Research Made Easy in
Complementary
and Alternative
Medicine

Cartoons by Kevin Macey

For Elsevier:

Publishing Manager: Inta Izols
Project Developmental Manager: Karen Morley
Project Manager: Jane Dingwall
Design Direction: Jayne Jones

Research Made Easy in Complementary and Alternative Medicine

Mark Kane MA DO ND MBAcC
Senior Lecturer, School of Integrated Health,
University of Westminster,
London

Foreword by
George Lewith MA DM FRCP MRCGP
Senior Research Fellow; Hon Consultant Physician
Complementary Medical Research Unit,
Royal South Hants Hospital,
Southampton

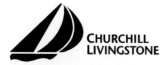
CHURCHILL
LIVINGSTONE

EDINBURGH   LONDON   NEW YORK   PHILADELPHIA   ST LOUIS   SYDNEY   TORONTO   2004

CHURCHILL LIVINGSTONE
An imprint of Elsevier Limited

First published 2004

ISBN 0 443 07033 4

British Library Cataloguing in Publication Data
A catalogue record for this book is available from the British Library

Library of Congress Cataloging in Publication Data
A catalog record for this book is available from the Library of Congress

NOTICE
Complementary and alternative medicine is an ever-changing field. Standard safety precautions must be followed, but as new research and clinical experience broaden our knowledge, change in treatment and drug therapy may become necessary as appropriate. Readers are advised to check the most current product information provided by the manufacturer of each drug to be administered to verify the recommended dose, the method and duration of administration, and contraindications. It is the responsibility of the licensed prescriber, relying on experience and knowledge of the patient, to determine dosages and the best treatment for each individual patient. Neither the publisher nor the author assumes any liability for any injury and/or damage to persons or property arising from this publication.
The Publisher

The publisher's policy is to use paper manufactured from sustainable forests

Printed and bound by CPI Group (UK) Ltd, Croydon, CR0 4YY
Transferred to digital print 2013

Contents

Foreword

As I read this book two ideas kept intruding into my concentration. The first was that I wished I'd had this text 25 years ago when I started developing research methodology in the field of acupuncture, and the second was the title. Why was such a text only relevant to complementary and alternative medicine?

Mark Kane has done a superb job, based largely on the teaching programme at Westminster, of systematising, defining and explaining a whole range of basic principles and concepts within the field of clinical research. He makes it clear in his introduction that the text is not exhaustive so those wishing to find a detailed understanding of statistical methodology will not find it here, but there are many other texts which explain this thoroughly. This text is targeted at undergraduates and postgraduates or those wishing to consider a research career. It explains the process of research superbly and defines methodologies that are entirely appropriate to the field of CAM. For instance, case control studies are not mentioned as they would largely be inappropriate to this field of clinical practice, however action research and individual case studies are considered in great detail, as appropriate, and indeed essential, techniques within CAM. In particular, the vexed question of systematic reviews is considered very carefully. Systematic reviews of inadequate and incompetent studies lead to either inappropriate or inconclusive interpretation of data. Negative interpretation of inconclusive data from systematic reviews has tended to bedevil CAM over the last 10 years and resulted in many substantial misunderstandings, and much inappropriate and misguided academic debate. The clarity of the chapter on systematic reviews therefore adds substantially to the literature in this area by placing their interpretation in context. If, as I suspect, this book will be used as primary course material for many of those wishing to study CAM disciplines at undergraduate level, then clarity of the issues and principles that govern the interpretation of systematic reviews in relation to good clinical practice will form an essential part of continuing professional development.

Thinking beyond CAM, however, this introduction to research would, in my view, serve as a superb introduction for anybody involved in considering research issues within any clinical discipline. It is as relevant to the medical, nursing, physiotherapy and occupational therapy undergraduate courses as it is to those studying CAM. It integrates an introduction to CAM research into the research disciplines of clinical medicine in a rigorous, thoughtful and yet suitably light-hearted manner with the addition of appropriate cartoons. It fills me with hope for the future. If we are training practitioners who understand these disciplines and would be looking at the practice of medicine through the thoughtful and critical principles of a disciplined research approach, then there will be a genuine dialogue between the osteopath, homeopath and GP with a shared understanding of scientific concepts. We may at last begin to speak the same language in a manner that will inspire a mutual respect.

I hope Mark Kane's book becomes essential reading, both at undergraduate level and through continuing professional development, at a postgraduate level, for all those within the field of CAM. It will serve as an essential introduction for anyone wishing to embark on a research career.

George Lewith
Southampton 2003

Acknowledgements

There are of course so many to whom I am indebted for all they have taught me from the great ancestors to my teachers, students, colleagues and patients. In particular I would like to express my gratitude to Mike Fitter, Phil Harris, Richard James, Hugh McPherson, Tessa Parsons and Veronica Tuffrey who provided helpful comments on draft chapters. This work would not have come about without the constant questioning by the masters students at the School of Integrated Health about designing research of relevance to practitioners which this book is an attempt to answer. The British School of Osteopathy supported my early work in research design. The editorial team at Churchill Livingstone/Elsevier have been highly supportive right from conception through to delivery.

My wife Simone and boys Finnian and Adam have been extremely patient whilst I was locked in the loft writing — thank you, I'm coming down to play now.

Mark Kane
London 2003

SECTION 1

Introduction

Introduction

1

BACKGROUND

The use of complementary medicine has mushroomed over the last decade. Along with the increased popularity there's been an increase in the number of practitioners who practise complementary therapies either as their primary discipline or as a 'complement' to their own discipline, such as nursing or medicine. With an increasing acceptance by the public and by mainstream healthcare professionals, practitioners of complementary medicine are being asked to provide evidence of the effectiveness and safety of their therapies. This is in line with a growing emphasis on evidence-based practice across all health-related disciplines.

Research into complementary medicine is still in its early days. Whereas practitioners of mainstream medicine have grown up in a culture of research, many complementary therapists have been educated in private teaching institutions outside of research-oriented universities, so these practitioners have had little exposure to practical research methods and the critical interpretation of research findings.

The economic constraints on private teaching institutions and individuals in independent practice have mitigated against the development of a research culture. Research costs money, and someone has to pay. For small institutions the imperative is to provide a sound education for their pupils; research is only an emerging priority. Most practitioners in the private sector — where most complementary medicine practice still takes place — do not have the funding, skills or organisational support to conduct successful large-scale research projects. However, with support and guidance it is possible for practitioners to conduct worthwhile studies.

QUESTIONING PRACTICE

There has been a degree of resistance to research from some quarters in the field. This resistance is in part based on the claim that complementary medicine emerges from a holistic philosophy and therefore is not amenable to the scrutiny of the scientific method, which is rooted in a reductionist philosophy. There is certainly an argument for using a wider range of designs than experiments in general and the randomised controlled trial in particular, but no justification for avoiding research altogether. The clinical trial can give precise answers to specific questions about effectiveness within a predetermined frame of reference. This, of course, presupposes that we know the right questions to ask and what parameters need to be evaluated— something that is certainly open to debate. Putting to one side ultimate questions about effectiveness, truth and the nature of reality, it seems to me that there are many valid questions that practitioners want to ask about their work — what it is they do in their practice and how they might do it better — that also deserve to be answered.

Knowing what patients believe about their health and illness, knowing how they value your treatment or other aspects of the care you give, establishing which patients and conditions you seem to manage most successfully, are all questions to which curious practitioners would like to have some answers. This is research that practitioners can engage in by themselves and for themselves.

WHY BOTHER?

All practitioners will have been in a position of needing to explain what it is they are doing in their work. The questions often come from patients who want to understand more about the treatment they are receiving. 'Will this treatment you are suggesting work?' 'How long will it take?' 'What sort of changes should I expect from having this treatment?' The more inquiring may ask: 'How does it work?' All are reasonable questions for patients to ask about the treatment they are receiving. Most practitioners will have learned to give answers to these kinds of questions. Their success in practice may well depend on their patients having an understanding of the approach being used.

Health professionals from other disciplines may also have questions about your work. 'Which particular complementary medicine treatments could help my patients and how would I be able to refer appropriately to complementary medicine practitioners?' 'Are the treatments safe?' They also may ask the question: 'How does it work?' Again, this is a reasonable set of questions to be asked by any practitioners thinking of referring their patients on.

Those responsible for increasing access to complementary medicine, whether they be legislators or purchasers of healthcare services, need to know that therapies are safe, effective and cost beneficial. To make such decisions on behalf of the public, a body of research is required.

Finally, all practitioners have a natural desire to know which of the treatments they offer to patients are most effective and they will have observed and noted, at least informally, the kinds of treatment that seem to be most beneficial in particular cases. Part of the duty and professional responsibility held by practitioners is to evaluate and improve the care they are offering to their patients.

WHAT IS RESEARCH?

Sometimes preconceived notions of what research is can put people off the idea of doing research. Images of laboratories, rats, white coats or endless questions in surveys come to mind. Whilst such caricatures do relate to certain kinds of research, there are also approaches to research that are much closer to what practitioners are already doing in their day-to-day work: looking, listening, trying new strategies and learning from experience. Research is really about being systematic and rigorous in how we examine our professional activity. It is my hope that the inquiring spirit underpinning good clinical practice can be applied more systematically to grow a body of knowledge serving those working in complementary medicine. Research should be useful for those in the field as well as for those called on to make judgements about it.

GETTING STARTED

This book is an attempt to provide practical guidance for students and practitioners of complementary medicine who want to inquire into their professional practice. It is not intended as a comprehensive treatise on the underlying philosophy or intricacies of each method; rather, the focus is upon actually getting a project started. Researchers will probably find that at some

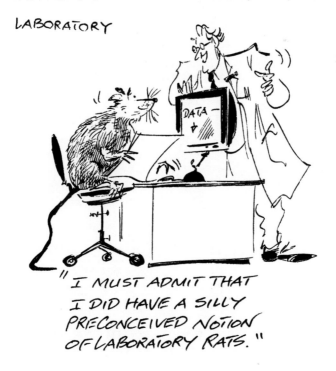

LABORATORY

" I MUST ADMIT THAT
I DID HAVE A SILLY
PRECONCEIVED NOTION
OF LABORATORY RATS. "

point in the project they will need to consult other works that give more detailed treatment of the specific methodology. The intention is to help researchers conceive and get off the ground inquiries relevant to their own fields of practice. The book provides the reader with a structure for formulating appropriate research questions, then describes a range of strategies and methods in terms of their working principles and the kinds of questions they are suited to answering. The advantages and limitations associated with each approach are then listed.

> ! *The aim of this book is to get you started on a project. It does not offer comprehensive coverage of the philosophy or intricacies of each method. You may need to refer to more specialist texts as the project develops and some pointers towards these texts will be in the reference sections of chapters.*

The student or practitioner looking at the prospect of doing some research may well feel trepidation in embarking on a project. OK, I'll come clean. The title of this book is a bit of an oxymoron: research is probably only rarely a straightforward affair. I would recommend you try to establish a network of support, both practical and emotional, to help you through what can sometimes be challenging terrain. I hope this book is able to guide the novice researcher in developing a project and avoiding some of the pitfalls and blind

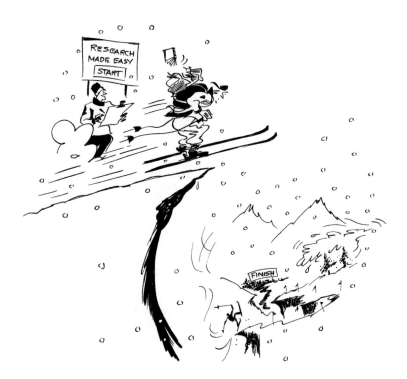

alleys. I can only speak for myself and many of the students I have tutored in saying that the research journey can be an exciting challenge with the potential to enrich the researchers' understanding of their own discipline. At the very least the traveller will have many tales to tell — so, bon voyage.

General design issues

2

WHERE DO GOOD RESEARCH IDEAS COME FROM?

Practitioners, whether they be novices or have years of experience, need only look at what happens in their clinical work to find a rich source of relevant questions. Ask yourself what it is that you do well with your patients and how that could be improved upon. All practitioners find within their practice certain areas where they seem to be especially effective, for instance the management of certain kinds of patients or conditions. Equally, they will recognise situations or cases that are much more of a struggle, for example interprofessional relationships or managing complex cases. Focusing either on what is going well or on areas where there are problems can be a very useful way to locate good research topics.

Well-formulated research questions do not normally appear out of the blue, they occur in the context of an existing body of knowledge. This context should be identified in a review of the literature and may include information about the biology, culture, epidemiology, public health importance, clinical relevance or current practice of the topic. This background helps set the rationale for the study, and should explain why the questions being asked are important.

IDENTIFYING THE TOPIC AREA

Don't worry if you don't have a precisely defined question to begin with – that can come a bit later. What can help at this earliest stage is to identify an area of your work in which there is a problem or puzzle you would like to solve. The problem or puzzle may not be clear initially, so you might begin by exploring an area of interest. It could be the treatment of children, or patients presenting with complex problems. Ask yourself some questions. What is it that makes this area interesting for you? What is the challenge for you in these situations? What do you already know about this area? How have you come to know this? By asking yourself how you know what you know, you are thrown back to the sources of your learning — teachers, books, experience. Examining your own experience as a practitioner is a valuable starting point for any investigation.

IDENTIFYING THE AIMS OF THE STUDY

Having found an area of interest to explore, it becomes necessary to think about the aims of the study. The aim is what you want to achieve — where you want to arrive at through doing the study. Possibly this will have a personal aspect as well as a professional one. This might be to give an account of your own approach to practice or to improve your management of a particular patient group or to improve the way you record clinical data.

GENERATING GOOD RESEARCH QUESTIONS

Defining the research question is one of the most important steps in an inquiry and so deserves time and attention. A good research question is one that can

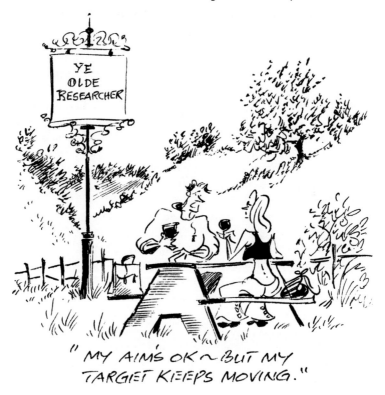

" MY AIM'S OK ~ BUT MY TARGET KEEPS MOVING."

generate some meaningful answers or at least a fruitful line of inquiry. Often first time researchers want to tackle very big questions. Does acupuncture lead to better health? Can homeopathy prevent acute illnesses from becoming chronic? Questions like these are certainly important, and they go to the heart of the claims made for complementary medicine, but the concepts used in the questions are so broad that a small-scale project is unlikely to be able to do justice to such questions. A concept like health has many dimensions and evaluation methods, such as morbidity, mortality, health-seeking behaviours and health beliefs (Bowling 1991, 1995). Without more specific terms of reference, a broad concept like health won't help you to reach meaningful conclusions about these kinds of questions. If, on the other hand, you are interested in what the word health means to a population of patients or practitioners, then it is perfectly valid and necessary to start with such a broad term. It all depends on the nature of the inquiry and whether you are trying to explore or confirm.

By making the aim of the research explicit you can begin to think about which methodologies would be appropriate to employ. A clear statement of the aim will guide your inquiry and be the basis of the specific research question that you ask.

PROVING OR IMPROVING

To demonstrate that a specific therapy or intervention is more effective than a placebo – which, by the way, can be extremely effective (Peters 2002) – the gold standard method in medical science is the randomised controlled trial (RCT). The organisation, sample size and time scale for an RCT make this kind of research unrealistic for students or small-scale practitioner-researchers. Exactly what makes the RCT the gold standard for outcome studies will be discussed in Chapter 8, Experiments and quasi-experiments. However, this does not mean that small outcome studies, evaluation of diagnostic methods or even single case studies are not worthwhile or that no meaningful conclusions can be drawn. Small-scale or pilot studies are often the important first step towards a full-scale clinical trial, but the findings tends to be suggestive of the methodological issues that should be addressed in the larger-scale study rather than establishing any firm evidence (White & Ernst 2001, White et al 2000).

Whilst it certainly is important to make sure that the claims we make for our therapies are valid, there are many areas of daily practice where the crucial concern is not to provide proof that what we do works, but to learn to improve what it is that we are doing (Fitter & Thomas 1997, Reid & Proctor 1995). The impetus to produce research that establishes the effectiveness of complementary therapies is often externally generated, whether by funding bodies, regulators, mainstream medicine or other groups. There are also questions practitioners would raise amongst themselves to do with refining how they practice (Higgs & Titchen 2001). If we want our research to serve us as practitioners, helping us to do what we do better, then this needs to be reflected in how the aim of the study is stated. The difference may be as simple as asking the following questions. Does acupuncture relieve pain in arthritis? What part can acupuncture play in the management of pain in arthritis? The first question demands a yes/no answer or, to put it more accurately, a probability of yes or no that would have to be established through an outcome study. The second question seeks to understand how acupuncture can be used, where in a strategy for managing pain it might best be employed, and what makes that so. It leaves ultimate questions of efficacy to one side. It starts with an assumption that acupuncture may have some part to play, but without predetermining what that part would be. This type of question demands a more exploratory or developmental approach.

Another area with direct relevance to clinicians is establishing the reliability of diagnostic techniques (White et al 2000). There are many diagnostic techniques used in complementary therapies, such as palpatory findings in bodywork or examination of the pulse and tongue in acupuncture, that have not been adequately researched (Coyle et al 2000, Nilsson 1995a, 1995b).

It is important not to try and make any single study fulfil an overly complex set of aims. By keeping the aim clear and the design simple, there is a much stronger chance of coming up with meaningful answers to the research question and fulfilling your aim.

TURNING YOUR AIM INTO A SPECIFIC RESEARCH QUESTION

If the aim serves as the guide to your research, then the specific research question you ask acts as the vehicle that drives you through the territory that you are interested in. Without a clearly formulated research question, reaching your aim may be well nigh impossible. It simply won't take you where you want to go. The aim of the study and the specific research question need to be very clearly linked. You should be able to turn a statement that describes the aim into a workable research question.

 A clearly defined question should specify the types of participants, if there is an intervention or exposure what kind it is, and the types of outcomes that are of interest.

As an example, your aim may be to *understand* why your patients choose you and your particular therapy so that you can work towards making a better match between what you provide and what your patients expect. The general aim of understanding could be made more specific by stating that you want to know about their motivations and expectations in coming to see you. Framed as a question this might be: 'What are the motivations and expectations of patients

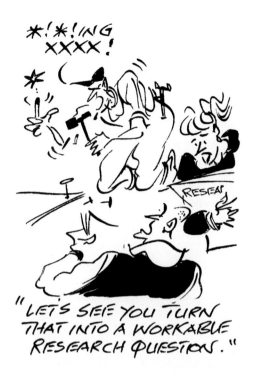

attending a homeopathy clinic?' or 'Why do patients choose homeopathy and
what do they expect from homeopathic treatment?'

 *A good research question is one that is answerable within the
confines of available resources.*

SETTING OBJECTIVES FOR THE RESEARCH

Once you have become clear about the project aims and have at least
tentatively settled on a question, the next step is to set your objectives. The
objectives are the actual steps to be taken to move you towards your aim. To
elaborate on the earlier example about why patients choose homeopathy
and what they expect from homeopathic treatment, the objectives might
be to:

1.   identify a sample of patients from the clinical records
2.   seek informed consent of the selected sample to be interviewed
3.   conduct a series of in-depth interviews
4.   explore within the interviews why patients chose to attend for
       homeopathic treatment, what they believed was the nature of their
       problem and in what way they thought homeopathy might help
5.   analyse the interview data to identify key themes
6.   write up results.

The objectives should identify what you will do to answer the question you have formulated.

THE CONCEPTUAL FRAMEWORK

The conceptual framework is made up of the theories you will use to help you research your topic. It is a set of propositions that define how you intend to approach the subject. You could think of it as a lens through which to look, a rationale and a set of principles for examining your topic. If you were interested in non-verbal communication between patients and practitioners, then the theories of as well as the methods for studying non-verbal communication would form the basis of your conceptual framework. The conceptual framework focuses the study and narrows down how you choose to conduct the study. It gives an indication of what will be included in the study and, equally importantly, what is outside the scope of the study. It marks the boundaries of the investigation. To extend the above example, you might be interested in the significance of non-verbal communication from a psychodynamic perspective – for instance, how unconscious drives find expression in the body. That would require a broader conceptual framework that included psychodynamic theories. The conceptual framework provides a basis for the specific questions you ask, what kind of data might be important to collect and the approach to analysis. In the ethnographic study of a chiropractic clinic (Cowie & Roebuck 1975), sociological theories of deviance and marginalisation guided the choices made in data collection and analysis (see the ethnography of a chiropractic clinic in Ch. 7, Ethnography, p. 67).

Try making your assumptions explicit

As you go through the stages of identifying the aims and objectives and the specific research question, the conceptual framework underpinning your work may become evident. Some people find they start with a specific question and then work backwards to specify their conceptual framework; others find it more helpful to start with some of the propositions and theories that they intend to utilise within the study, then move towards a specific question. You may find it helpful to work back and forth between the theories (conceptual framework), the questions and the aims of the study.

All studies are based on assumptions; however, these are not always stated. Take, for example, the assumption that it is possible to know about the world in an objective way. The concept of objectivity underpins what is known as 'scientific method' and a range of specific methods and techniques have been elaborated to work with this assumption, such as placebo interventions and blinded observers in experiments. There are also assumptions about procedures and their validity and reliability. In scientific research objectivity is a fundamental concept and is not normally discussed except in the methodological literature. Most scientific studies simply report what specific strategies and measures were adopted to maintain objectivity, but not all studies assume or

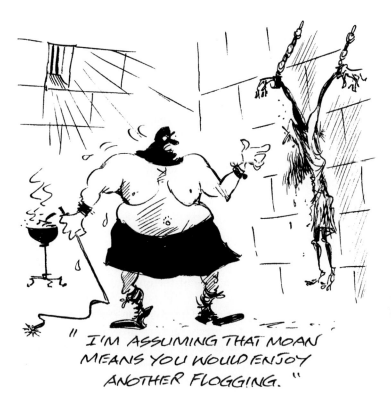

" I'M ASSUMING THAT MOAN MEANS YOU WOULD ENJOY ANOTHER FLOGGING. "

aim for objectivity (Denzin 1997). For instance, there are approaches to research that emphasise the subjective nature of human experience (Moustakas 1994).

Emic or *etic* perspective?

Part of your conceptual framework is the position you adopt in relation to your research topic. If you intend to develop an insider's understanding and interpretation of the topic, as in some interview or case study work, this is known as the *emic* perspective. The *emic* perspective attempts to preserve the integrity of the insider's view and presents the world using the insider's own words and categories for ordering that world. The *etic* perspective utilises theoretical constructs that are external to the individual or group being studied in order to gather data, analyse and present interpretations of that individual or group. The *emic* and *etic* positions are poles of a continuum and your project may draw on both perspectives. For further elaboration on this see the section on the *emic/etic* perspective in Chapter 14, Observations.

By making your assumptions explicit you can demonstrate why the approach you have chosen is a valid one and that any claims you make for your research are anchored within the parameters of this set of guiding assumptions (Higgs & Titchen 2001). It is not a defect of qualitative research methods that they rely on the subjectivity of participants, but any claim for validity would have to acknowledge that the findings are not an objective account.

Although it is important to make some explicit statements about the theories and assumptions your study rests upon, this does not mean you need to spend most of your study defining every assumption, but you should be able to set out in a few paragraphs the underlying structure of the study and what sort of knowledge you are trying to generate.

WHICH METHODOLOGY SHOULD I USE?

When the aims, the question and the conceptual framework are defined, the units of analysis become clear. The nature of the question will suggest the appropriate methodologies. There needs to be congruence between the question that is asked, the position adopted by the researcher and the methodology chosen. If you want a precise answer to a specific question, such as whether acupuncture is more effective than anti-inflammatory drugs for pain relief in low back pain, an outcome study would be the logical choice.

To devise a methodology that is appropriate for your project it may be helpful to classify the purpose of the research. You could think in terms of whether the project is descriptive, exploratory, explanatory, interpretive or developmental.

It may be:
- **Descriptive:** e.g. providing an account of your current practice or a set of events (Pringle & Tyreman 1993).
- **Exploratory:** e.g. asking what happens when complementary practitioners attempt to establish collaborative working relationships with orthodox practitioners (Emanuel 1999, Paterson & Peacock 1995).
- **Explanatory:** e.g. proving or disproving a clearly identified hypothesis such as 'Does a homeopathically prepared antigen have a greater effect than placebo in patients with hayfever?' (Reilly et al 1986).
- **Interpretive:** e.g. asking what meanings we can attribute to emotional states in chronic illness (Klienman 1988), or how therapists make sense of patient disability (Mattingly 1991).
- **Developmental:** e.g. establishing and refining appropriate referral criteria for complementary therapies (Peters et al 2002), or developing an outcome measure for holistic practice (Long et al 2000).

Of course many studies do not fall neatly into the category of being descriptive or hypothesis testing and may have elements that are both interpretive and developmental, but classifying the purposes of the research will help in choosing the most appropriate methodology.

Qualitative or quantitative?

There is a tendency when describing qualitative and quantitative research to refer to them as polar opposites. It is certainly true that in scientific research great value is put on objective quantifiable data that can be statistically manipulated. The methods favoured in some branches of the social sciences are more qualitative and interpretive, but that does not mean the different forms of data are mutually exclusive. For very good reasons science has favoured the use of objective data to help researchers take account of certain kinds of bias. For equally good reasons social scientists, with their interest in the opinions, feelings, interpretations and behaviours of human beings, have developed sophisticated and refined ways of gathering and analysing qualitative data. There is not much to be objective about when analysing feelings or opinions, but that does not mean that the interpretation of such data is not open to other kinds of scrutiny or

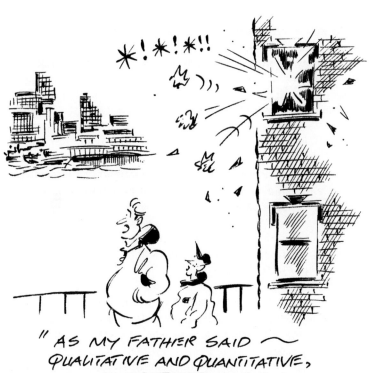

" AS MY FATHER SAID ~
QUALITATIVE AND QUANTITATIVE,
NEVER THE TWAIN. "

validation. There is an ongoing discussion about researchers using a combination of qualitative and quantitative methods and there are some examples of where these have been successfully applied (Oths 1994). Case study research, in particular, favours the use of multiple data sources and methods of analysis. The important point is to allow the choice of methods to be dictated by the research aims rather than by adherence to a particular methodological orthodoxy.

WRITING A PROJECT PROPOSAL

Having defined the aim of the research and a research question, it becomes essential to develop a workable plan for the project. This should include mapping out all the crucial steps you will need to take to see the project through to final completion, including writing the project up − an important part of the research that consolidates your learning.

When research is to be part of a dissertation project there is normally a requirement formally to present a proposal for approval by the research coordinator and possibly by a full research ethics committee. If patient care is to be altered, the approval of a research ethics committee is a requirement. Each committee will have its own format for the presentation of the proposal (see Ch. 4, Research ethics).

As well as often being a formal requirement, writing a research proposal obliges us to make very clear statements about the purpose, aims and methods of the study we intend to initiate. It may be possible to remain vague and ambiguous in discussions about the project, but when it comes to committing ourselves to writing we really need to have a clear sense of how the project will hang together, both conceptually and practically.

The plan should include all the stages that you intend to go through to finish the project, including formulation, execution and reflection. Many of the difficulties encountered throughout a project relate to the design and planning stage. A great deal of attention should be given to mapping out both where you want to get to and how you intend to get there. This can be mapped out as a flow chart (Fig. 2.1) showing the series of steps you will take to bring the project to completion. For each of the stages identified, try to specify where, when and who will take responsibility for each step.

It is also useful to create a project timetable (Fig. 2.2) that will lay out when you intend each stage of the project to take place. At the very least this is important for research review panels and ethical committees and for negotiating access to your chosen research site. It is also a great help in ensuring that the project is on track and that you are not getting endlessly bogged down in planning and reviewing the literature.

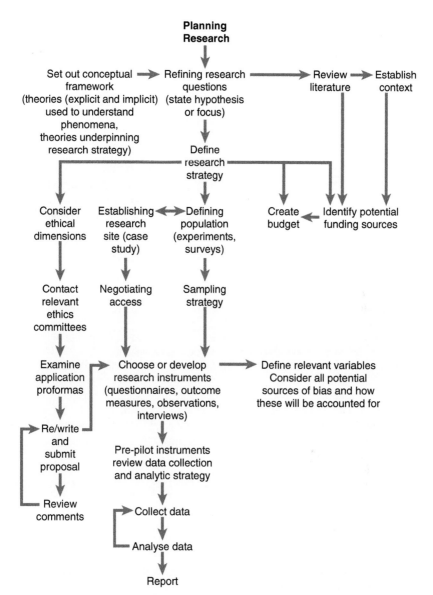

Figure 2.1   Planning research.

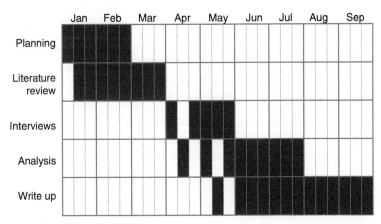

Figure 2.2 Project timetable.

References

Bowling A 1991 Measuring health: a review of quality of life measurement scales. Open University Press, Buckingham

Bowling A 1995 Measuring disease: a review of disease specific quality of life measurement scales. Open University Press, Buckingham

Cowie J, Roebuck J 1975 An ethnography of a chiropractic clinic. The Free Press, Macmillan, New York

Coyle M, Aird M et al 2000 The cun measurement system: an investigation into its suitability in current practice. Acupuncture in Medicine **18**(1): 10–14

Denzin N 1997 Interpretive ethnography: ethnographic practices for the 21st century. Sage, Thousand Oak

Emanuel J 1999 Will the GP commissioner role make a difference? Exploratory findings from a pilot project offering complementary therapies to people with musculo-skeletal problems. Complementary Therapies in Medicine **7**: 170–174.

Fitter M, Thomas K 1997 Evaluating complementary health care for use in the National Health Service. Horses for Courses Part 1: The design challenge. Complementary Therapies in Medicine **5**: 90–93.

Higgs J, Titchen A 2001 Practice knowledge and expertise in the health professions. Butterworth Heinemann, Oxford

Kleinman A 1988 The illness narratives: suffering, healing and the human condition. Basic Books, New York

Long A, Mercer G et al 2000 Developing a tool to measure holistic practice: a missing dimension in outcomes measurement within complementary therapies. Complementary Therapies in Medicine **8**: 26–31

Mattingly C 1991 The narrative nature of clinical reasoning. The American Journal of Occupational Therapy **45**(11): 998–1005

Moustakas C 1994 Phenomenological research methods. Sage, Thousand Oak

Nilsson N 1995a Measuring cervical muscle tenderness: a study of reliability. Journal of Manipulative and Physiological Therapeutics **18**(2): 88–90

Nilsson N 1995b Measuring passive cervical motion: a study of reliability. Journal of Manipulative and Physiological Therapeutics **18**(5): 293–297

Oths K 1994 Communication in a chiropractic clinic: how a DC treats his patients. Culture Medicine and Psychiatry **18**(1): 83–113

Paterson C, Peacock W 1995 Complementary practitioners as part of the primary health care team: an evaluation of one model. British Journal of General Practice **45**: 255–258

Peters D 2002 The placebo response in complementary and alternative medicine. Churchill Livingstone, London

Peters D, Chaitow L et al 2002 Integrating complementary therapies in primary care. Churchill Livingstone, London

Pringle M, Tyreman S 1993 Study of 500 patients attending an osteopathic practice. British Journal of General Practice **43**: 15–18

Reid J, Proctor S 1995 Practitioner research in health care: the inside story. Chapman & Hall, London

Reilly D, Taylor M et al 1986 Is homoeopathy a placebo response? Controlled trial of homoeopathic potency, with pollen in hayfever as model. Lancet **ii**: 881–886

White A, Ernst E 2001 The case for uncontrolled clinical trials: a starting point for the evidence base for CAM. Complementary Therapies in Medicine 9(2): 111–116

White A, Williamson J et al 2000 A blinded investigation into the accuracy of reflexology charts. Complementary Therapies in Medicine 8(3): 166–172

Reviewing the literature

3

ESTABLISHING CONTEXT

Before embarking on any research project it is important that you get to know the current literature in the field. You may not have been the first person to consider the question that you are proposing. Even if your research question is novel it is important to ground your study within the relevant literature.

AVOID RE-INVENTING THE WHEEL

Previous studies can highlight difficult and unfruitful research areas within your chosen subject area. Understanding what other researchers have concluded can help you to refine your own research question so you can avoid having to re-invent the wheel. Even Einstein said that we stand on the shoulders of giants in his acknowledgement of the work of scientists like Newton. Your work should grow from your own curiosity and the stimulation provided by the work of others. It may be that someone has studied one aspect of your topic or used slightly different methods. Understanding what others have done can help you to identify a new angle or niche that has yet to be explored.

BALANCING BREADTH AND PRECISION

With the plethora of books, journals and electronic media in every discipline one could easily spend months and years immersed in the literature, but it is important to ensure your search has sufficient breadth and depth. The literature sources and the kinds of studies you identify as relevant probably need to be wider than the precise question in your specific discipline.

In the first phase of literature searching it is important to keep your search wide. Only when you have located significant source material and have gained a feel for this literature will you begin to narrow your focus. It may be that there is an abundance of literature relating to your question. You will soon identify common themes, questions and concerns. Understanding what others in your field are concerned about helps you to place your own research questions within a context. If you are unable to identify sufficient literature you may need to widen the net of your search in the literature of related disciplines, but sometimes it is more a question of searching smarter than going further afield.

SMARTER SEARCHING

Current texts

An easy place to start identifying the concerns and questions within the discipline is to scan current texts by leading-edge authors. Even if textbooks

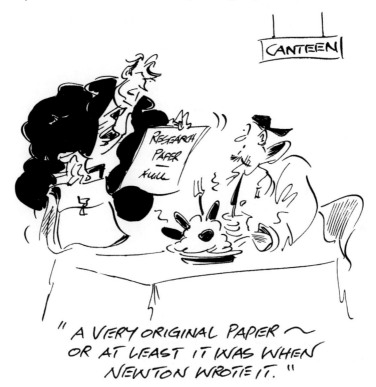

" A VERY ORIGINAL PAPER —
OR AT LEAST IT WAS WHEN
NEWTON WROTE IT. "

sometimes present their material without posing critical questions, the reference sources should be helpful in getting to know who's who and what kind of work they are doing. Books dedicated to research in complementary medicine, such as Ernst 2001, Ernst & Hahn 1998, Ernst & White 1999, Lewith et al 2002, and Vincent & Furnham 1997, can be useful resources to identify some of the methodological debates and published research.

Web-based searching

There are numerous ways of sourcing literature via the web, such as using a good general search engine like google.com. More specific are databases such as PubMed (MEDLINE). PubMed, the largest medical database, is available online without charge. There are many other specialist databases and some of these may be available online via subscription. University or health service libraries will usually subscribe to a range of online databases and these can be accessed if you have some affiliation with the University or health service.

DEFINING THE SEARCH STRATEGY FOR LOCATING RELEVANT STUDIES

When searching databases such as PubMed, include multiple key words to ensure that you do not miss studies. If you are interested in the treatment of neck pain by osteopathy, as well as using the key word neck pain you should also include cervical spine pain. As well as using osteopathy you should also include manipulation, physiotherapy, chiropractic and manual medicine. By using the word 'or' between the above words you will locate any papers containing these key words. The 'Boolean' logic of this kind of search strategy is built into most databases. You will refine this further by using the word 'and' with key words such as randomised controlled trials, clinical trials, placebo. A very short example of a search strategy follows in Box 3.1. In practice the 'ands' and 'ors' may be much more elaborate that the example here. Searching databases comprehensively is a science in itself, and expert input from specialist librarians or others skilled in this is recommended.

Box 3.1 A simple search strategy

(Neck pain **or** cervical spine pain **and** osteopathy **or** manipulation **or** physiotherapy **or** chiropractic **or** manual medicine) **and** (randomised controlled trial **or** clinical trial **or** placebo controlled trial)

CITATION INDEXES

Another way of tracking relevant literature is by doing a citation search. This is where you identify a key paper and then search for other papers that have included this key paper in their references. Online bibliographic services such as SCISEARCH and BIDS perform this specific function very simply. You may turn up unexpected leads that would not be obtained from one of the bibliographic databases such as PubMed and gain an impression of the importance of particular papers by seeing how widely they are cited.

Searching subject-specific databases such as PsychINFO for psychosocial studies and the databases of the Research Council for Complementary Medicine (CISCOM) or the British Library (AMED) for research in the field of complementary medicine is likely to identify many studies not found on PubMed. Box 3.2 lists useful resources for web-based searching.

Box 3.2 Useful resources

Available without subscription:
- PubMed is the US National Library of Medicine database, at www.ncbi.nlm.nih.gov/PubMed/
- The UK National Electronic Library for Health is located at www.nelh.nhs.uk

Through bibliographic services such as BIDS (subscribed to by academic institutions) full-text articles or abstracts can be obtained by searching databases such as:
- AMED, hosted by the British Library or ALT-HEALTHWATCH, contains abstracts and full-text articles in the field of complementary medicine
- CINAHL is the nursing and allied health database
- PsycINFO links to abstracts and full-text articles in psychology, psychiatry, sociology, anthropology
- CISCOM, hosted by the Research Council for Complementary Medicine, contains a very extensive citations and abstracts database. A fee is payable for each search. www.rccm.org.uk/ciscom

---

Hand searching

There may be specialist libraries in your field that you could visit and hand-search for relevant publications. As with all forms of searching you are likely to find diminishing returns for your search efforts and just how much time you can spend doing this will depend upon deadlines and available resources. The specialist librarians may be able to help point you towards the relevant publications.

Identify literature in related fields addressing your question

If you cannot find any work related to your research question within your own field, you may need to look to a related discipline where the questions you are asking have already been explored. For instance, the use of audit has been well developed for more than a decade in medicine but only recently has its use become commonplace in the complementary medicine field.

Bibliomania and knowing when to stop searching

You must know when to finish your active search of the literature. When every search of the databases or libraries produces diminishing returns and you have a fairly good feel for what's going on in the field, it is time to move on. Bibliomania — the endless search for that vital paper to complete your literature review — is one way to ensure your project never gets completed. Typically, time constraints and deadlines oblige researchers to move onto the next phase of their work and this is not always a bad thing. You can of course go back to the literature at a later stage to address specific queries in light of your findings.

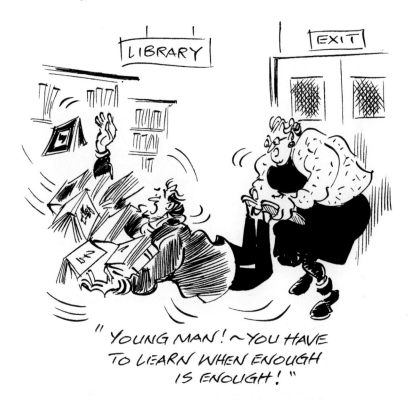

" *YOUNG MAN! — YOU HAVE TO LEARN WHEN ENOUGH IS ENOUGH!* "

IF YOUR RESEARCH QUESTION HAS NOT BEEN ASKED BEFORE — CHECK WHY

Perhaps you have not been able to locate literature relating specifically to your proposed topic. This may mean that your research topic is novel and yet to be researched or it may imply that others in the field have not considered the issues you are intending to explore either relevant or researchable. A good research question should help you move towards a greater understanding in your professional work and be sufficiently specific so that meaningful conclusions can be drawn. Even if you are moved by the really big questions like 'What does my life as a practitioner mean?' or 'Does my therapy work?' you will need to ensure your current project is broken down into manageable bits.

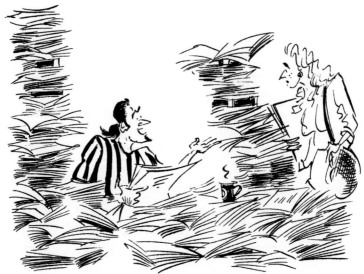

" I'VE BROKEN THE MANAGEABLE BITS
INTO MANAGEABLE BITS ~ AND YOU'RE
LOOKING AT THE MANAGEABLE BITS
OF THOSE MANAGEABLE BITS. "

HOLDING A CRITICAL PERSPECTIVE

Holding a critical perspective is about maintaining a healthy degree of scepticism and not taking what others have said or written for granted. It also refers to the process of carefully analysing the arguments and evidence for what people say.

It is important to approach the literature with a critical perspective. Just because something exists in writing we should not assume it to be true. We need to identify the basis of claims made and evaluate them to see whether they are justified. There are various devices other than reason and research evidence that can be used to persuade readers.

Some common fallacies in arguments

APPEALS TO AUTHORITY

The authority of an eminent personage may be called upon so that we might trust their judgement rather than make our own. This appeal to authority is the same as when celebrities endorse products in advertising. It relies on the persuasiveness of the personality rather than evidence and argument.

CHARACTER ASSASSINATION

The antithesis of the above is when an argument is dismissed by discrediting the author. Whilst this approach is widely used in TV courtroom dramas, a

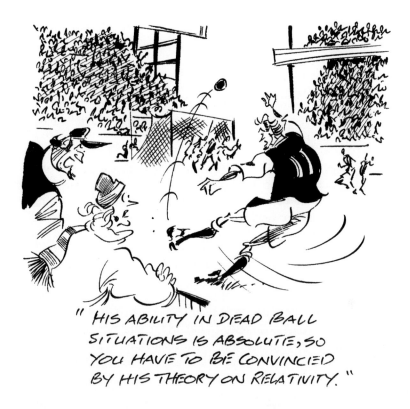

" HIS ABILITY IN DEAD BALL
SITUATIONS IS ABSOLUTE, SO
YOU HAVE TO BE CONVINCED
BY HIS THEORY ON RELATIVITY. "

character assassination is not the same thing as seriously addressing the content of an argument.

APPEALS TO TRADITION

Calling on tradition is another device used by some authors. The fact that acupuncture has existed for thousands of years is not proof of its efficacy any more than the fact that child slavery has been around for millennia is proof that it is natural and a good thing. Each claim must be evaluated on its own merits. If a tradition or practice has existed for centuries it clearly must be fulfilling some need and is an area worthy of investigation, but this should not be confounded with proof of the claims made.

Look for coherence between the research question, method and conclusions

Consider whether the methodology is suited to answering the question being posed by the research. At one level this might be quite obvious — a survey will be unable to provide definitive proof of the efficacy of a treatment. Surveys are designed to canvas opinions and beliefs. An experimental method such as the randomised controlled trial is the method of choice for establishing that one treatment is more effective than another (within defined parameters), but it provides little information on the opinions, beliefs and behaviours of a population (unlike interviews, questionnaires and observational research).

Another area in which to be critically aware is the conclusions drawn from any single piece of research. It is not too uncommon to find authors extrapolating extravagantly from their findings and making far-reaching recommendations regarding changes in practice, policy and funding, e.g. more funding should be put into their field of interest.

Peer-reviewed journals offer some help in that experts critically review submitted papers. That said, all publications have their own defined area of expertise and are guided by the perspective of the editor. For instance, not many qualitative research studies are published in the *Lancet* and, equally, experimental studies are unlikely to end up in *Social Science and Medicine*. The editors and reviewers of the different journals act as gatekeepers to the kind of research that gets published (Resch et al 2000). Most of the prestigious publications in medicine favour quantitative research, although in recent years some journals such as the *British Medical Journal* have signalled a shift in attitude by regularly publishing qualitative research studies. Nursing literature tends towards qualitative research but, as the qualitative–quantitative debate runs its course through the different disciplines, there is a growing recognition of the distinctive contribution that each method can provide, with articles

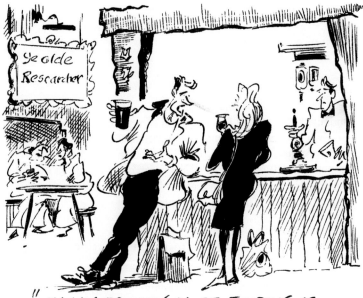

"IN MY OPINION MORE FUNDING IS NEEDED IN MY FIELD OF INTEREST ~ BUT UNFORTUNATELY MY RESEARCH DOESN'T BACK ME UP."

being published according to their relevance rather than according to methodological prejudice.

DIFFERENT KINDS OF LITERATURE

There are various kinds of source material you may draw on to develop your inquiry. Each has its own rigour and criteria to be judged by. You need to be clear about how to evaluate and use these different kinds of work, which are listed in Box 3.3.

Box 3.3 Different kinds of literature

- **Research** includes experimental studies, case studies, surveys, cohort studies, sociological studies and epidemiological studies.
- **Conceptual** literature offers frameworks for understanding phenomena. Using different underpinning assumptions can vary the meaning given to different facts.
- **Methodological** literature establishes appropriateness for inquiry.
- **Reviews** provide a survey of the field.
- **Current textbooks** can give a feel for the opinions, attitudes and practices that have currency in the field.
- **Grey literature** refers to publications that have not been widely disseminated in the public domain, including reports, dissertations and official publications.

Identify the gaps in the literature

Sometimes it is difficult to formulate your own question precisely. It can seem as though all the important lines of questioning have been identified by other authors and the best you can do is to try and answer their questions. By surveying the literature you can become aware of where the gaps in knowledge lie. These gaps are what we do not know, and if your curiosity is drawn into the shadows then the puzzles they present can provide an impetus for your own research.

Springboard for your own inquiry

Sometimes novice researchers can lose their own unique perspective when they read the erudite and persuasive work of other authors. It is important to understand the work of others to contextualise your own work, but equally important not to suppress your own original thought. Clarify the links between the question you are asking and how it relates to your field of practice and, importantly, what really motivates you to inquire. Your own curiosity can be an invaluable source of steam to drive your project to completion and you let it escape at your peril.

Try to stay clear about your own research question — avoid being enchanted by the words of other authors.

References

Ernst E 2001 The desktop guide to complementary and alternative medicine. Mosby, London

Ernst E, Hahn E 1998 Homeopathy: a critical appraisal. Butterworth Heinemann, Oxford

Ernst E, White A 1999 Acupuncture: a scientific appraisal. Butterworth Heinemann, Oxford

Lewith G, Jonas W et al 2002 Clinical research in complementary therapies. Churchill Livingstone, London

Resch K, Ernst E et al 2000 A randomised controlled study of reviewer bias against unconventional therapy. Journal of the Royal Society of Medicine 93: 164–167

Vincent C, Furnham A 1997 Complementary medicine: a research perspective. John Wiley & Sons, Chichester

Research ethics and ethical committees

4

INTRODUCTION

The basic tenet of ethical research is to preserve and protect the dignity and human rights of all participants in a research project. These rights are enshrined in the Declaration of Helsinki (1964, amended 2000) and have been elaborated by research funding bodies such as the Medical Research Council in the UK and the Australian National Health and Medical Research Council. In the US the National Research Act (1974) led to the development of guidelines for human research in the biomedical and behavioural fields (National Commission 1979).

With the increased recognition of the potentially harmful effects of research, it is now routine practice for a researcher to gain ethical approval before a study is commenced. It is an institutional requirement of universities and hospitals as well as many funding bodies. The major medical and health-related journals have made ethical approval for the research a prerequisite for publication.

Most academic institutions and hospitals conducting research will have an established process for reviewing research proposals. In the UK all research conducted within the National Health Service (NHS) must be approved by a designated ethics committee for the local region (LREC) in which the study takes place. For research on NHS patients from widely dispersed geographical regions there exists a raft of regional ethics committees (Multi-centre Research Ethics Committees or MREC) that can act in a national role to obviate gaining approval from each and every local ethics committee that might be involved in a multicentre or geographically spread study. There are variations on this in the US and Australia and most institutions will have established guidelines on the procedures.

In those instances where research is being conducted independently of institutional ties the researcher should still seek to have the proposed project evaluated by a research ethics committee. Some associations or bodies governing professional practice have a process for evaluating proposals in relation to their field. There is widespread recognition that individual researchers should not bear the responsibility for being both the judge and jury of the ethics of their proposed research. The membership of the ethics committee should represent expertise that includes medical, legal and research ethics as well as lay or user representation. The role of the ethics committee is to consider each project's ethical and practical dimensions. The first of these dimensions is the potential for harm and benefit (Royal College of Nursing UK 1998).

THE PRINCIPLE OF NO HARM

Harm can be physical, psychological or social. The risk of harm must be evaluated by the researcher as well as by the ethics committee and the guiding principles are that the risks of participation must be no greater than would occur in routine practice (in a clinical setting) or that participants would encounter in their normal lifestyles (field setting). Any foreseeable risks should be identified and the procedures for minimising risk and managing any adverse events clearly stated. This should include insurance against damage that occurs as a result of participation in the research project. Institutions such as universities and hospitals normally insure themselves against such risks. Independent

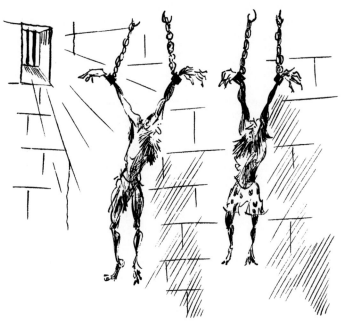

" IF I'D KNOWN WHAT WOULD HAPPEN
I'D NEVER HAVE GOT INVOLVED IN THIS
RESEARCH PROJECT. "

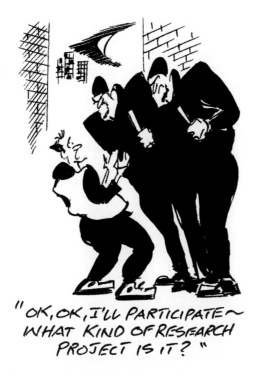

"OK, OK, I'LL PARTICIPATE ~
WHAT KIND OF RESEARCH
PROJECT IS IT?"

researchers will need to look carefully at what coverage they may be able to secure through their professional bodies.

It is also for the researcher and the ethics committee to evaluate the potential benefits of the research to the participant and/or the wider community. The degree of risk, however minimal, needs to be seen in relation to potential benefits. Individuals agree to participate in research for a wide variety of reasons. Most healthcare research would not take place but for the goodwill and desire of participants to do something that will alleviate human suffering. In respecting the autonomy and free will of individuals to make their own choices, the principle of informed consent is the next key area to be evaluated.

INFORMED CONSENT

Part of the respect for individuals' autonomy and freedom to make their own choices is that the decision to participate in a research project is an informed one. That is, they should know what they are getting into. Participation can be at many levels. In an action research project the participants will have significant input into the design, implementation and reporting of the study. In survey and experimental research the main input of participants may be simply filling in a questionnaire or agreeing to be assigned into a group receiving experimental treatment. Whatever the level of input, it is important that participants understand why the research is being conducted (in broad terms may be adequate), what is expected of them, and any risks they may be undertaking.

Wherever practical, informed consent should take the form of a written statement explaining the purpose and scope of the study. The actual wording will depend on the specific project but will include a description of the procedures, what is expected of the participant, any known risks and how they will be managed should such an occurrence take place. There must be a clear statement that participation is voluntary and the decision not to participate or to withdraw at any time during the study will not prejudice the participant in any way. Also included should be a point of contact for further queries (such as the telephone number of the researcher) and the name of any supporting institution. A signed copy of the consent form should be collected prior to the participant entering the study.

With some research designs such as postal or telephone surveys it is not usual to have a written consent form. The fact that the questionnaire has been returned, or the agreement to answer questions on the telephone, is taken as consent to participate. There should of course be appropriate explanations of the relevant ethical dimensions, such as an explanation of the purposes of the study and that confidentiality will be respected.

Informed consent in naturalistic studies

Seeking informed consent in a formal study such as an experiment is often comparatively straightforward. The boundaries are made quite explicit in the research design. There is a clear beginning and end to the experiment. There are explicit recruitment procedures in which all potential participants are given full information about the study. They may opt to join the study or not. On the other hand, many real world designs such as ethnography, action research and observational studies do not have such clearly defined boundaries spelling out who is in and who is outside of the study. Clearly an observer collecting data on a street corner could not ask each person he observes for consent, much less to sign a consent form allowing the observer to use the data. The participant observer in a large organisation would not normally be expected to gain full informed consent from each and every person that he encounters or observes. Apart from the practical difficulties of seeking each and every person's consent, the naturalness of the situation would be disturbed. In studies where the observer is a full participant, his identity as a researcher might be unknown to most of the participants. The observed behaviour may well differ when people know they are being observed. However, these practical and methodological difficulties do not exempt the researcher from working within ethical guidelines. The researcher and the ethics committee should be satisfied that any individuals in a real world study who are not asked for consent will not suffer as a result of their being observed. Also their privacy should be respected by ensuring anonymity and confidentiality in reporting.

Although these principles are easy to state, there may be cases where information gathered by the researcher could be used against those observed in the study. For instance, the organisation supporting the study may use the findings as ammunition to hire or fire staff, or to fund or drain resources from the area the researcher has studied. Researchers need to be conscious that their findings may be used in ways they had not intended.

There are some approaches to research where seeking the active participation of all those with a stake in the research is a guiding principle. In action research the intention is to research *with* people rather than *on* them. The level of participation given by all stake holders is an important criterion of the validity of the research (see Ch. 5, Action research).

Vulnerable groups

Another special consideration is that some individuals may not be in a position to give full and informed consent. These vulnerable groups include children, elderly people, mentally disabled people, those with psychological disturbances and patients with severe or terminal illnesses such as cancer. An ethics committee will examine very carefully whether a study including such participants can be justified on the grounds of potential benefit and whether there are sufficient safeguards in place to ensure that the participants' human rights are not compromised by the research.

Inducements, deception and coercion

Sometimes inducements are offered to participate in research, including rewards of money, access to health care or other payments in kind. The ethical principle that must be considered is that the reward should not induce participants to take risks beyond what is normal for their lifestyle. Inducements can be problematic in other ways. Research participants are well known for telling researchers what they believe the researcher wants to hear (regardless of requests not to do this) and inducements can increase the sense of obligation participants feel to give the right answers. One way around this is **deception**, such as not revealing the specific hypothesis or focus of the study, but deception conflicts with another ethical requirement, i.e. giving fully informed consent, and will not generally be condoned by ethics committees unless there are extraordinary arguments in favour and specific safeguards in place. A related ethical concern is that there should be no **coercion** to participate. This can be problematic when the participants are already in some kind of relationship to the researcher or to those responsible for recruitment. For example, patients, students or junior colleagues may feel an obligation to join a study. The pressure to participate may not be made explicit but can be real none the less. The researcher should be satisfied and should make explicit that no prejudice or alteration in participants' usual relationships (e.g. patient, student) will occur should they decide not to participate or indeed if they choose to exercise their freedom of choice and withdraw from the study.

The right to withdraw from the study

It should be made clear (normally in writing) that any participants are free to withdraw from the study at any time and this will not prejudice them in any way. This is especially important for vulnerable groups (whether they be children, elderly people or other institutional captives such as patients, students or inmates) who might feel that their continuing level of care, support, progress or well being is contingent upon pleasing their practitioners, teachers or carers.

PREPARING A SUBMISSION FOR AN ETHICS COMMITTEE

Each ethics review body will have its own requirements in terms of documentation and will usually provide a proforma with the relevant categories. These include:

- Research question and rationale
- Recruitment procedures – inclusion and exclusion criteria
- Inducements
- Potential for harm and benefit
- Procedures for protecting against harm and minimising risk
- How informed consent is gained
- Procedures for ensuring privacy (anonymity and confidentiality and conforming with the Data Protection Act) (see Ch. 18, Writing up).
- Data collection and analysis.

Committees will be very keen to see exactly what patients are being asked to sign up for in research studies, so they tend to scrutinise very carefully patient information leaflets and consent forms, often being very particular about the wording. Questionnaires to be used in the study are likewise required for vetting. As well as the obvious ethical dimensions of harm, risk and privacy, the committee will also want to be satisfied that the methodology of the research is sound. They will want to be sure the research question is clear and the design is suited to answering the question. It is unethical to waste participants' time if the study is unlikely to generate useful data and the analytic procedures are not matched to the data and research question. The goodwill of individuals to participate in research is not inexhaustible and should not be wasted on projects that are unlikely to generate meaningful data due to poor methodology.

You should be prepared for the fact that it can take several months for approval to be granted as many ethics committees meet only monthly or less frequently (ask for their schedule of meetings and submission dates). Committees frequently return proposals with queries and suggestions for revision and the researcher will need to answer those queries and sometimes

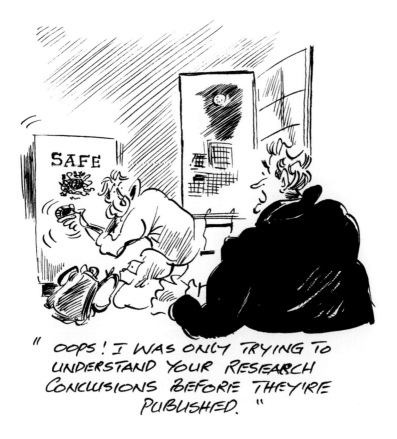

" OOPS! I WAS ONLY TRYING TO UNDERSTAND YOUR RESEARCH CONCLUSIONS BEFORE THEY'RE PUBLISHED. "

rework the proposal in time for the next meeting (Chair's action is sometimes taken to approve minor changes). Your research timetable should take account of the fact that gaining ethical approval for a study can take several months.

The degree of scrutiny by the whole committee depends upon the level of risk posed by the study. Low-risk studies may be exempt from this formal review, for example in a retrospective study of clinical records when data collection is part of normal practice. Most institutions will have criteria and a screening process to establish by whom your proposal should be considered. If no screening process is in place you should seek advice from your local ethics committee about whether or not a full submission is required.

Approval is usually granted for a specified period of time and the committee may require a report if there has been a significant change to the study design or, in longer-term studies, an annual progress report.

The process of submitting your proposal to an ethics committee can be a bit daunting. There may be long lists of questions and a requirement to submit multiple copies of your proposal (for distribution to committee members), as well as the possibility that the proposal may not be approved without changes.

If the study is geographically dispersed, there may be a requirement to gain approval by more than one committee. But these procedures are the price the research community pays for ensuring the protection of participants and the continuing support of the wider community for health research.

References

National Commission 1979 Report of the National Commission for the Protection of Human Subjects of Biomedical and Behavioural Research (the Belmont Report). The National Commission, Washington

Royal College of Nursing UK 1998 Research ethics: guidance for nurses involved in research or any investigative project involving human subjects. RCN Publishing Company, London

US Congress 1974 National Research Act

World Medical Association 2000 Declaration of Helsinki (revised)

SECTION 2

Strategies

Action research

5

WHAT IS ACTION RESEARCH?

Under the broad banner of action research lie a number of related approaches. These include cooperative inquiry, participative action research and reflexive action research, to name a few. These approaches share a commitment to bringing about practical change to real world problems. The strategy may be applied to the individual, as in reflexive action research (Rolfe 1998), or to the community, as in participative action research (Lewis 2001). Cooperative inquiry has frequently been used by groups of professionals wanting to improve their practice (Reason 1994).

CHARACTERISTICS OF ACTION RESEARCH

Practical research

Action research emphasises the issues and concerns of practice over the development of propositional theory. The focus is on bringing about change in specific situations rather than developing propositional knowledge. The knowledge that is developed is specific for the context rather than generalisable.

A concern frequently voiced by practitioners is that the findings of published research too often have insufficient relevance to day-to-day practice. The distinctive feature of action research is its emphasis upon the practical, problem-solving dimension of research. While there may be practical applications from all forms of research, action research makes problem solving the goal of the inquiry. This does not mean that there is no theory developed in action research, but the theoretical developments stay close to the concerns of practice. The approach has a broad appeal to groups of people wishing to address their shared concerns and

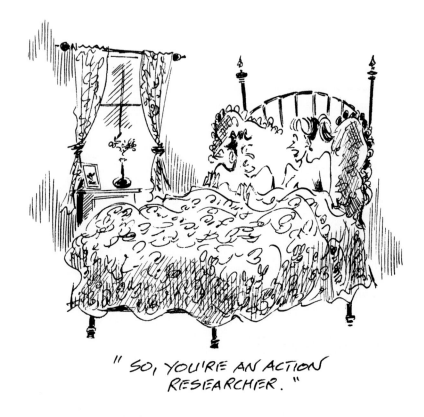

" SO, YOU'RE AN ACTION
RESEARCHER. "

to practitioners disenchanted with the ability of scientific research to address practical problems. The strategy has been utilised in fields as diverse as medicine, management, nursing, community and social work and complementary therapies (Reason & Bradbury 2001).

The action researcher's aim is to bring about change and evaluate the impact of that change in the real world. Research in this sense is not seen as an additional activity but as an integral part of practice — akin to the form of reflective practice described by Schön (1983, 1987). Drawing on their own or the group's tacit knowledge of the issues and problems, researchers modify their current activity, introduce innovations and then critically examine the outcome of these innovations. This moving back and forth between action and reflection is crucial in order to ground theoretical developments in the world of action and reformulate action strategies in light of emerging theory. The characteristics of action research are described in Box 5.1.

Cyclical process

This is in contrast to the ideal of the scientific method, in which the researcher is in a detached and distant position with a predefined hypothesis to be proven

Box 5.1   Characteristics of action research

- Problem focused and context specific
- Theory development subservient to solving practical problems
- Participative: traditional divide between researcher and researched broken down. Researcher as facilitator rather than detached observer
- Researching *with* people rather than *on* people
- Cyclical process of action, reflection, reformulation of problem, action
- Practical know-how of participants is valued along with propositional knowledge

or disproven. Scientific researchers use their distance and detachment to limit bias creeping in. By contrast, action researchers set out to examine rigorously what it is that is currently going on in their practice, then introduce modifications and observe the result — not from a distant and detached position, but from the coal face of practice. In working through iterative cycles of action and reflection, the practitioner/researcher finds new and creative ways of viewing and addressing problems.

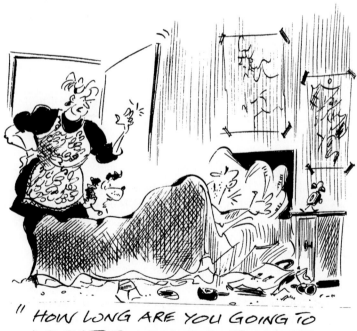

" HOW LONG ARE YOU GOING TO WORK THROUGH THE ITERATIVE CYCLES OF REFLECTION STAGE BEFORE GETTING TO THE ACTION? "

The approach does not ignore the fact that we can be seduced by our own perceptions and introduce bias. Action research has developed a number of ways to take into account these selective perceptions. By working through cycles of action and reflection in collaboration with others, it is possible to view our experiences from a variety of perspectives. We can challenge our own and others' interpretations and look for evidence that these claims are based on actual experience. For this to take place effectively, the group needs to build in processes that ensure the inquiry is genuinely collaborative and takes into account the voices of all participants. In reflexive action research practitioners challenge their own perceptions by drawing on different data sources, both objective and subjective.

Participation

Another characteristic feature of action research is the commitment to encouraging participation in every stage of the research process. It is sometimes described as research *with* people rather than *on* people. This willingness to take account of the experience and perspectives of the participants and to engage them in the research is part of the democratising principle underpinning action research. This bottom-up approach encourages participation in setting the agenda for the research, engaging in cycles of inquiry and deciding how the findings of the research should be used. This is enormously validating and empowering for participants, who may not be expert researchers but who have experience and a personal stake in the area of study. The role of the expert researcher is de-emphasised and participants' knowledge and experience are brought into the foreground.

The aim of going through cycles of action and reflection is not simply to come up with a set of findings that can be written up; rather, through a process of learning, those involved become better equipped to deal with the practical issues. This educational or developmental aspect to research is one of the strengths of action research.

Ownership and empowerment

Another foundation of the participative approach is that the research ought to belong to those who stand to lose or gain from it. This contrasts with the classic scientific stance, where the crucial decisions about the research are in the hands of the researchers rather than in the hands of the subjects of the study. The rationale is that detachment is required to prevent bias creeping in, but the effect of this detachment can be alienation from the inquiry process. If those who stand to lose or gain from the research are excluded from the decision-making processes, then they are unlikely to feel that the findings 'belong' to them — often a crucial factor when it comes to implementing changes and applying the findings of research.

Professional researchers answering questions generated within the framework of their own speciality may not be addressing the issues that concern practitioners or patients (Higgs & Titchen 2001). The question becomes one of who has the right to name and categorise the issues? A crucial aspect of the validity of action research is ensuring real participation of all those involved in the inquiry — in the questions that are asked, in the methods chosen, and in how the results are used. It is sometimes assumed that the outcome of proper research should be learned papers written in professional journals. Whilst this is no doubt of value, action research emphasises bringing about change in practice. It sees the ultimate purpose of theory as being to guide and assist practice, empowering those involved with the research to become active participants in bringing about change in their environment and working practices.

Researcher as facilitator

Rather than being the detached investigator, the researcher's role is one of facilitator and networker in the process of helping the group formulate their interpretation of the situation and problem, in negotiation and consensus, handling conflict and monitoring change. For this to take place successfully, all those who have a stake in the inquiry and its outcomes need to be contacted. Researchers who are outsiders may find they are not automatically accepted in this role as facilitator and only through a process of negotiation and consensus is the legitimacy for this role gained (Heron 1996).

Practitioner knowledge

Action research is built on the premise that you can't study human experience by stepping outside of it; or if you do, you risk losing some crucial aspects of the experience, i.e. that which is unique and individual that you bring to the experience — yourself.

In response to the particular demands of their work situation, practitioners develop their own unique and idiosyncratic ways of solving problems. The expertise of practitioners is only partly based on their formal education. In developing expertise practitioners learn to apply those principles in ways that fit the demands of their local situations. This expert practitioner knowledge is sometimes described as an 'art'. Because of its idiosyncratic nature and the difficulty in describing what it is, practitioner knowledge is rarely researched, in spite of being at the heart of good practice (Higgs & Titchen 2001, Reid & Proctor 1995).

Action research, with its iterative cycles of action and reflection, is suited to exploring and developing this kind of knowledge and practical expertise. Through this process, practitioner knowledge can be validated as well as challenged and improved. This developmental approach to research has found a place in fields such as education (Whitehead 1989), nursing (Hills 2001) and complementary therapies (Peters et al 2002a, see Example 5.1).

Example 5.1 Action research (Peters et al 2002a)

Since the late 1980s the Marylebone Health Centre has been working on the issue of integrating complementary therapies into an NHS primary care setting. Since the first research projects of the early 1990s (Reason 1991, Reason et al 1992), ongoing cycles of action, reflection and evaluation have been maintained through regular clinical, team and academic meetings and a common focus upon the collaborative nature of integrated health care.

The most recent documentation of this ongoing research is published in Peters et al (2002a). In particular, the chapter 'Delivering and evaluating the service' describes how these action research cycles have underpinned the development of the provision. The chapter 'Reflecting on and adapting the service' documents some of the lessons learned along the way.

Aims
- To establish an effective service integrating complementary therapies into NHS primary care with a built-in capacity for learning about the difficulties inherent in multidisciplinary collaboration.
- To establish a criteria-based set of guidelines for GP referral to the in-house complementary therapy service that would meet the identified needs of the practice.

Design
A series of four cycles were initiated:
1. Needs identification
2. Mapping intake and expectations
3. Evaluating complementary therapy referrals and the practicality of using outcome measures as part of daily clinical work
4. Tracking and evaluating patients through a series of consultations

Each phase of the research required different methodologies. The first phase, **identifying needs,** was based on questionnaires, discussion of available research evidence and consensus development. The second phase, **mapping intake and expectations,** was based on a retrospective study of the previous year's complementary therapy referral forms. These documented the conditions GPs actually referred for and their expectations from the referral. The lists of conditions from phase one and two, along with a collation of the evidence base for complementary therapy treatment, led to the development of guidelines for GP referral.

In the third phase, **evaluating referrals and outcome measures,** the practicalities of using a structured outcome tool were evaluated through an analysis of the MYMOP (see Ch. 8, p. 84) referral form and semi-structured interviews with a sample of patients and all practitioners who had filled in the forms.

The fourth phase, **tracking and evaluating patient outcomes,** led to refinements in the implementation of MYMOP and the development and piloting of a clinical database.

In addition to the weekly meetings exploring organisational and interprofessional issues, where many of the issues raised by the research were explored, there were also bi-monthly research meetings, where members of the clinical team discussed the emerging questions and progressed the project.

Outcomes

In action research the aim and validity criteria rest on the ability to bring about improvements in the field of practice. In this case the provision of a needs-led quality-assured service was the aim. Peters et al (2002a) documented in detail the background to the study and the process and methods used, as well as lessons learned along the way. In addition, a set of educational guidelines for designing and evaluating complementary therapy service provision was created. These guidelines formed the basis of Marylebone Health Centre's own evaluation, one arm of which has shown that it is possible to establish appropriate frameworks and supportive interprofessional processes that allow a more integrated approach to practice (Peters et al 2002b). Further action research cycles have illustrated that it is no easy task to mould the daily professional practice of a multidisciplinary group. Even after its structures and processes have been jointly developed and are effectively co-owned, it takes time and continuing effort to make full use of them and to close learning loops.

AN EXTENDED EPISTEMOLOGY

Peter Reason (Reason 1994) has described how different forms of knowledge are integrated into the action research process. Heron (1996) provides a framework or 'extended epistemology' to explain this. We have our own *experience* which is a form of knowledge. This is our face-to-face meeting with our work. Before we rationalise and put our explanations and theories onto what is happening in our work, we experience the world 'as it is'. This provides the ground for other forms of knowing. *Presentational* knowledge is in the form of imagery or symbols that we use to express our experiential knowing. From that we build *propositions* or theories to explain our experience. *Practical* knowing is the skill or competence we gain, having absorbed the three prior forms of knowledge — experiential, presentational and propositional.

The purpose of describing this 'extended epistemology' is to indicate that the outcomes for our research may well be in any of these knowledge domains. A cooperative inquiry will pass through these different domains in a cyclic process: direct experience–symbols and imagery–theory–skills or expertise. This is, in fact, a key method to ensure that research findings are valid within a cooperative inquiry: taking our experience; finding ways to give expression to or symbolise that experience; making statements or propositions about that experience, i.e. theorising; and finally the acquisition of particular skills or expertise which are then grounded back in the world of action and direct experience (Fig. 5.1).

GENERALISABILITY

Because the focus is on solving concrete problems, it may be difficult to generalise the findings from one piece of action research to other settings. Each particular problem is context bound, and the action research process is directed to addressing these specific issues. In this respect there is a parallel with case studies, which have as their focus a single site or instance. The ability to generalise from this very specific and context-bound research depends on the similarity in important characteristics, and is described by Yin (1994) as analytic generalisation, as apposed to statistical generalisation. This means establishing the similarity and transferability on a case-by-case basis (see Ch. 6, Case studies) and requires that the reporting of the action research project is in sufficient detail or 'thick description' to allow this comparison.

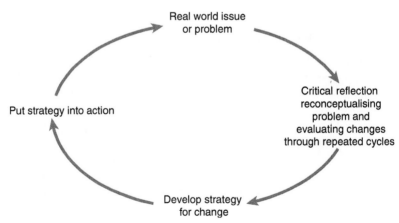

Figure 5.1 Action research cycle.

ADVANTAGES

✔ A practical method to bring about change that facilitates learning for individuals and groups

✔ For practitioners there may be no need to establish a research site. The site of ongoing practice is the site for the research

✔ Practitioners can use the strategy to improve their own practice

DISADVANTAGES

✘ Because a central feature of action research is problem solving within a specific context, generalising the findings to other contexts may not be so easy

✘ Difficult to apply — practitioners struggle to get time for critical reflection, and the factors that shape current practice are often the result of complex social and political forces or resource limitations that make change beyond the reasonable expectation of practitioners

References

Heron J 1996 Co-operative inquiry: research into the human condition. Sage, London

Higgs J, Titchen A 2001 Practice knowledge and expertise in the health professions. Butterworth Heinemann, Oxford

Hills M 2001 Using co-operative inquiry to transform evaluation of nursing students' clinical practice. In: Bradbury H (ed) Handbook of action research: participative inquiry in practice. Sage, London, p 340–347

Lewis H 2001 Participatory research and education for social change: Highlander Research and Education Centre. In: Bradbury H (ed) Handbook of action research: participative inquiry in practice. Sage, London, p 356–362

Peters D, Chaitow L et al 2002a Integrating complementary therapies in primary care. Churchill Livingstone, London

Peters D, Harris G, Pinto G 2002b Using a computer-based clinical management system to improve effectiveness of a homeopathic service in general practice. British Journal of Homeopathy **89** (suppl 1): S14–19

Reason P 1991 Power and conflict in multidisciplinary collaboration. Journal of Complementary Medical Research 5(3): 144–150

Reason P 1994 Participation in human inquiry. Sage, London

Reason P, Bradbury H 2001 Handbook of action research: participative inquiry and practice. Sage, London

Reason P, Chase D, Desser A et al 1992 Towards a clinical framework for collaboration between general practitioners and complementary therapists: discussion paper. Journal of the Royal Society of Medicine 85: 161–164

Reid J, Proctor S 1995 Practitioner research in health care: the inside story. Chapman & Hall, London

Rolfe G 1998 Expanding nursing knowledge: understanding and researching your own practice. Butterworth Heinemann, Oxford
Schön D 1983 The reflective practitioner. Temple Smith, London
Schön D 1987 Educating the reflective practitioner. Jossey-Bass, San Francisco
Whitehead J 1989 Creating a living educational theory from questions of the kind: How do I improve my practice? Cambridge Journal of Education 19(1): 41–52
Yin R 1994 Case study research design and methods. Sage, Thousand Oaks

Case studies

6

WHAT IS A CASE STUDY?

Case studies are often chosen by researchers doing small-scale projects who want to investigate some aspect of the real world. The appeal lies in the flexibility afforded to researchers to adapt their inquiries to the contours and demands of real people and situations. Unlike experiments, which require the researcher to be able to control the environment and important variables, the case is typically studied as it exists in the real world, without attempting to introduce changes. That does not imply that case studies are soft on rigour — far from it — but they require a particular approach to rigour that can take into account the complexities in which most cases are embedded. The study is in-depth, with a focus upon the circumstances, dynamics and complexity of a single case. Case study describes a strategy for research rather than a specific method. What makes this approach distinctive is the commitment to *study things in the context in which they naturally occur*. This empirical approach to research deals with complexity by favouring the use of multiple methods and data sources to tease out the case details and to cross-check findings to ensure their validity. The characteristics of case study research are listed in Box 6.1.

> ### Box 6.1 Characteristic of case study research
>
> - Focus on the particular, whether an individual, organisation, event, process
> - Selection of a single case or small number of related cases rather than large samples
> - Illuminate the general by looking at the particular
> - Detailed and in-depth study
> - Focus on relationships and processes and how the parts interrelate rather than on outcomes
> - Case is seen in context
> - Naturalistic setting, unlike experiment where the researcher introduces variables and the conditions are controlled
> - Multiple methods and data sources are used in order to investigate in-depth complex situations and to validate the findings. This cross-checking process is known as triangulation
> - Data sources include: observation, interviewing, videotapes, reviewing artefacts. Documentary evidence can be important, including patient records, minutes of meetings, reports, assessment reports

Seeing the particular – in context

Case studies are also distinctive in their *focus on the particular* – whether that be an individual, an organisation or an event. Sophisticated sampling techniques have been developed in survey and experimental research to reduce the significance of the unique and particular, and to ensure that the sample chosen for the research is representative of the wider population. The findings of properly conducted surveys or experiments can be confidently generalised to the population in question. Cases studies are not chosen from a representative sample and each case is treated as unique. The sampling strategy is purposive rather than representative (see Ch. 11, Sampling). The case is the unit of study, rather than the population. This is the strategy of choice when we want to learn from individual instances, whether they be patients or aspects of clinical practice, management or policy (Luff & Thomas 2000). Surveys and experiments limit the number of variables under investigation, but case studies are useful when it is not clear which variables are important and the boundaries between the phenomenon we are studying and the context in which it occurs are not clear. To quote Yin (1994, p. 13): "you would use the case study method because you deliberately wanted to cover contextual conditions – believing that they might be highly pertinent to your phenomena of study."

Multiple methods

Another characteristic feature of case studies is their use of multiple research methods and data sources. The focus is upon depth rather than breadth. By using multiple methods and data sources it is possible to cross-check and corroborate findings, supporting the validity of the findings by building up a web of evidence. In surveys and experiments findings are validated by cross-checking them with a representative population. This contrasts with case studies, where an intricate picture of the evidence is built up by establishing the cross-linkages and relationships *within* the case rather than checking to see whether the same findings exists for other people in the population (Fig. 6.1). Both qualitative and quantitative methods can be used in case studies.

Focus on relationships and processes

A strength of the in-depth view developed in case studies is that the relationships and processes within the case and between the case and its context can be studied. Rather than focusing on isolated factors, the emphasis is on how the different parts interrelate. In this respect case studies can give a holistic account of the hows and whys of the case rather than giving just the end-point or outcome (Luff & Thomas 1999). For instance, if you were evaluating a complementary therapy provision within a primary care unit, a structured questionnaire could be used to establish the level of satisfaction with the service. The findings might indicate that the service is highly regarded by users, but the results from a user satisfaction questionnaire alone would not tell us what was going on *within* the service that made the users rate it so highly. It could be the seamless care from referral to making appointments and being seen promptly, or the high-quality care from the practitioners, or even the fear that the service might not be continued if the users rate it poorly. A case study would explore the detailed workings that make up the service by using a range of methods such as interviews, observations and records. These could be integrated with the findings of the questionnaire to develop a more complete picture.

CASE STUDIES AND THEIR USES

Case studies are widely used in a variety of disciplines where experimentation and limiting an investigation to a few pre-specified variables would be inappropriate. For instance, anthropology has developed a particular approach

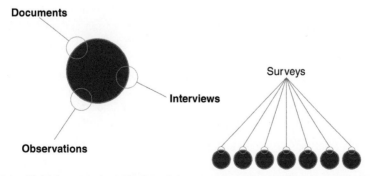

Figure 6.1   Multiple research methods and data sources of case study, compared with survey which gathers the same kind of data from a sample of the total population.

to case study called ethnography, in which the implicit rules and customs within a culture are described and analysed (Farquhar 1991). Case studies have also been used to explore innovations in practice (Luff & Thomas 1999). Case studies are much used as a teaching tool but this should be differentiated from case study as a research strategy. For teaching purposes the case need only stimulate discussion and debate, and the accuracy of empirical data may be willingly sacrificed to highlight a point — not an acceptable stance in research.

To explore or explain

Case studies can be used to explore or to explain. If you wanted to know the requirements for the successful implementation of a new technique or innovative service, then an exploratory case study would be a useful strategy that could be reported as a set of recommendations for practitioners and policy makers (Luff & Thomas 1999). The purpose of an explanatory case study is to build an explanation for events with a raft of evidence gathered from multiple sources. The researcher builds a compelling case for the chosen explanation, presenting the evidence and demonstrating the robustness of the explanation by posing competing explanations for the same events and then arguing why the chosen explanation is the most convincing (Borckardt 2002).

Flexibility

The flexibility that case study allows in the design and data-gathering phases enables the researcher to make modifications at a strategic and practical level. This could be in terms of what falls within the bounds of the case and the kind of data that should be collected. This helps the researcher shape the inquiry to the contours of the case. However, maintaining a flexible stance is not the same thing as having no idea what you are investigating or why. Even the loosest form of inquiry is informed by a set of general questions, assumptions and values and it is important that the researcher makes these explicit. Without clear statements to guide the inquiry, it is impossible to know what data should be included or excluded. Although flexibility is a valued characteristic of case study research there is no intrinsic reason why a tightly pre-structured approach cannot be taken. The crucial matter here is that all the data sources as well as the methods of collection and analysis are clearly defined — as is typical in surveys or experimental work. It may be advantageous that the researcher has a clear brief and can avoid being side-tracked. The disadvantage is that potential sources of valuable data discovered on the job cannot be included. The degree of flexibility or pre-specification depends partly upon why the study is being undertaken. Box 6.2 lists the choices that need to be made in designing a case study.

N=1

Whilst most case studies focus on relationships and processes and how the parts interrelate, rather than on outcomes, one type of case study called N=1

> **Box 6.2** Choices in case study design
>
> - Level — individual, event, service, organisation
> - Type — loose, pre-structured
> - Approach — exploratory, descriptive or explanatory
> - Methods — interviews, observation, documents
> - Analysis — holistic, embedded

does evaluate outcomes (Reuther & Aldridge 1998). These are sometimes known as single subject (or case) experimental designs or time series studies, and they are discussed in Chapter 8, Experiments and quasi-experiments.

HOW TO DEVELOP A CASE STUDY

Defining the case

In the real world where the case is embedded in its context, defining the boundaries of the case may not be obvious. It is important that you be explicit about what you consider to be *in* and *out* of the case. If you were interested in how an individual with cancer made use of self-help strategies, the case boundary would be at the individual level; but if you were investigating an outpatients' service designed to promote self-help strategies for cancer patients, then the boundaries may be less self-evident and you would need to set them in relation to the research question. In this example the boundary might be all the activities taking place within the physical environment of the health centre, but you would need to be clear that this was not excluding some significant activity taking place outside the centre. Where the boundaries are set has important implications for the data collection. The wider the boundary, the more expansive the data collection exercise becomes. It is also worth thinking about how your work would relate to any similar case studies in the literature, as this may be helpful in how you establish boundaries for the case. If you intend to make comparisons with other work, you will need to be clear in which ways the work might be similar as well as different, in particular, at what level the analysis is to take place, whether individual, group, event, service or organisation.

The research question

There is a relationship between the research question and how the case is defined. The way the question is framed should give some indication of the case and its boundaries. The question must also be linked to the conceptual framework.

How the research question is framed and the conceptual framework that is used will guide you in setting the boundaries of the case. You may start with only the broadest notion of your research question, or you may have a precise question that you want to answer. Either way, you will need to map out your conceptual framework to *ensure there is consistency between the research question, the conceptual framework and the methods you will use to carry out the study* (see Ch. 2, General design issues).

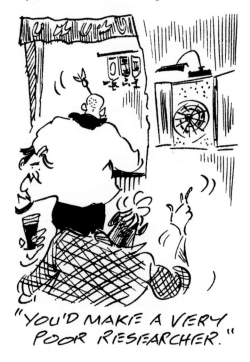

"YOU'D MAKE A VERY POOR RESEARCHER."

The conceptual framework

The conceptual framework is the set of assumptions and principles (explicit and implicit) that orient you in the inquiry. These may come from your own experience or from theory and research from your own discipline or another field. For instance, if you were a nurse using aromatherapy you might be interested in exploring the value of aromatherapy in a geriatric ward. Your conceptual framework would have to include your definitions of nursing, geriatrics and aromatherapy as well as the kinds of benefits or value that you would be looking for. Making some of these guiding assumptions explicit helps to refine the research question and ensure internal consistency. Chapter 2, General design issues, explores how you develop your research question and conceptual framework. You may well find yourself having to return to these issues as the shape of the inquiry begins to consolidate. It can be helpful to map your understanding of the conceptual framework and your research question by putting it in a simple diagram.

Sampling strategy

As discussed in Chapter 11, Sampling, choosing a case is not done on a random basis or to be representative of a wider population. The choice is purposive because you believe the distinctive features of the case are worthy of study in their own right. You could say that each case comes from a population of one, or in multiple case studies from a series of cases with shared characteristics in which each case is investigated in its own right. Certainly there may be an element of convenience or serendipity in how you choose the case. For many small-scale researchers the workplace, or some activity, process or individual within it, may present itself as the most appropriate case. This is more than a question of convenience — a poor basis by itself for selecting a case. The researcher will know the workplace and the current issues, as well as potential data sources, and is likely to be in a good position to gain access to the data. Negotiating access to patients, staff, documents or even to a site for observation may be extremely difficult for an outsider and at best is likely to take considerable time. The disadvantage of investigating a familiar site is that it is difficult to factor out our prejudices and see the situation afresh, but this needs to be weighed against the benefit of an insider's understanding of the situation. There are various ways of taking account of the bias inherent in being an insider or an outsider. Wherever one is situated, the perspective is bound to be different from that of those situated differently. What is important is that these biases are not left unexamined.

Single or multiple case designs

Researchers need to give thought to whether their designs will be single or multiple case. When the case you have chosen is a one-off event or an individual with a rare condition, the choice is self evident. It may be that you have access to a type of case for which there is little theory or explanation, and a single case study could explore and explain aspects of this case. The single case design may also be appropriate when you want to test the fit of a theory to a particular case. The case might confirm, challenge or extend the theory (Borckardt 2002).

A multiple case design can be used to compare and contrast cases or to replicate findings in a series of cases. The cases are analysed in their own right, and not gathered together as a sample for a general analysis as in surveys. The analysis is based on theories of the phenomena which may be confirmed, challenged or extended. Luff & Thomas (1999) analysed 10 separate cases individually and then did a thematic analysis and mapping exercise of the 10 case studies in terms of general issues (see Example 6.1).

ANALYSIS OF CASE STUDIES

It is important to be clear about the level at which analysis is to take place. Yin (1994) differentiates between what he calls *holistic* and *embedded* case studies. His definition of a holistic case study is where the analysis takes place at a single level. This approach is useful where no logical sub-units can be

Example 6.1 Case study research (Luff & Thomas 1999, 2000)

Luff and Thomas (1999, 2000) looked at different models of complementary therapy provision currently being used in primary care settings. They wanted to know what needs the schemes were expected to meet and how these were working in practice. Funded by the Department of Health in the UK, the report was designed to inform policy makers of the issues in integrating complementary therapies within primary care.

Aim

Through a series of case studies they aimed to:
- Give a descriptive analysis of 10 purposively selected schemes
- Assess the perception of impact of the scheme within each organisation
- Identify the benefits, problems and pitfalls with general relevance in implementing complementary therapies in primary care.

Conceptual framework

While no explicit conceptual framework was articulated in the report, it is clear from the aim that the innovational nature of the organisational dynamics was guiding the research structure, interview schedules and analysis of the data.

Sampling

A sampling frame was created based on a survey of complementary therapy provision in primary care as well as identifying centres through published literature. Eighty-seven centres were identified as offering current provision. From this 87, 13 practices were purposively selected based on criteria such as how established the complementary therapy service was, typical as well as innovative forms of provision, low-profile as well as high-profile practices, those asking for some form of payment and those which did not. Ten out of 13 selected practices agreed to participate.

Multiple methods were used including:
- Semi-structured interviews with key informants
- Critical incident reviews
- Review of exisiting records relating to service
- Simple audit form for the complementary therapy practitioners to use
- Direct observation for 2–4 days within each practice.

Interview schedules with key informants were designed to gather data on:
- Rationale and perceived need
- Organisational features
- Patient management — how access to the complementary therapy service is controlled and how decisions about who gets access, continuation of care and discharge are arrived at

- Clinical management – referral strategies
- Integration of the complementary therapy practitioners – how boundaries are maintained and how conflict is managed
- Impact of service – perceived effect of the service on the practice as a whole
- Future developments.

A small number of patient interviews were conducted using a critical incident approach to explore issues of accessibility, acceptability and perceived appropriateness.

Analysis
Transcripts of the interviews were summarised. A preliminary coding framework of themes was identified based on concerns identified in the planning of the study.

Each practice was viewed as a separate case and data for each case were collated.

Contradicting as well as similar data in each case were explored to produce a nuanced account of each practice.

These separate case studies were the basis of thematic charting, mapping and interpretation of the whole data set in the search for category and pattern generation and testing of the emerging hypothesis.

Reporting
The full case report published by the Medical Care Research Unit who carried out the study for the Department of Health is a 178-page document. Aspects of the study were also published in *Complementary Therapies in Medicine* (Luff & Thomas 2000).

The full report concentrates on a description of each case and a more general analysis in terms of perception of benefits and constraints to integration, with discussion and recommendations for policy makers. The report concludes with three appendices detailing the methodology used, an analysis of the service users' perspective and a preliminary audit of costs. As is typical for reports prepared for policy makers, the methodology section did not elaborate greatly on what informed the overall thematic charting, mapping and interpretation.

identified and the research question is concerned with the global level rather than the inter-working of the parts. For example, if you were studying an individual patient and how she manages in her environment, it may not be necessary to break the analysis down into sub-units because you would be interested in how your case – the individual, as a global entity – was relating to her environment. In an embedded design the analysis is divided into levels.

If you were evaluating how effectively a service was meeting the demands of its users, it might be meaningful to analyse your case — the service — by breaking it down into the different sites at which the service is provided, different aspects of the service and different user groups of the service. It is important to *ensure that the level of analysis is appropriate for the research question and the case.* This means that in choosing a holistic design you need to be clear that there are no important sub-units of analysis being left out. In an embedded design the researcher needs to make sure the analysis does not stop at the sub-level without returning to the case as a whole.

Generalising from a case study

The question arises as to whether it is possible to generalise the findings of a particular case to a wider population. In contrast to statistical generalisation commonly used in surveys, case studies rely on what has been described by Yin (1994) as analytical generalisation. The confidence in *statistical generalisation* is based on the principle that the chosen sample share characteristics of the population from which they were drawn, therefore findings from the sample can be extrapolated to this population. *Analytical generalisation* depends on establishing the degree of similarity between different cases and settings. This needs to be done on an individual basis. Because an in-depth understanding of the case is developed, it becomes possible to make comparisons with other cases. Some of the relevant dimensions to compare might be physical, social, historical or contextual. Take a case study evaluating the impact of introducing complementary therapies within a general practice. To generalise the findings to another setting one would need to look at how comparable the practices were. If the practice in the case study was an inner city health centre serving a multi-ethnic population, with six GP partners and an extended team who met regularly to discuss clinical issues, then the applicability of findings from such a practice to a single-handed rural GP practice would be in question. What is important is to identify the significant features of the case for comparability. This requires the reporting of the case to have sufficient detail to allow the reader to make such judgements.

Triangulation

Having multiple data sources can be useful to corroborate findings. When more than one data source or more than one type of data are used to corroborate a particular finding, this is called triangulation. The validity of any findings is enhanced by this process. It may be that the different forms of data or data sources do not corroborate but challenge a particular finding. This does not automatically invalidate the results, but the researcher will then need to explain why this contradictory finding exists. This may require a revision of current theory to account for the difference, or it may challenge the validity and application of the research methods.

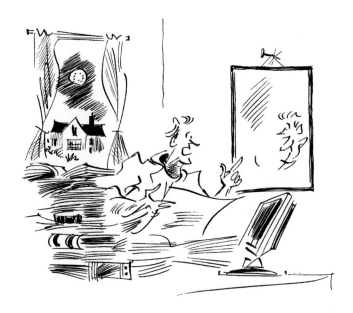

" IF IT WASN'T FOR YOLI CORROBORATING MY RESEARCH I'D GO INSANE. "

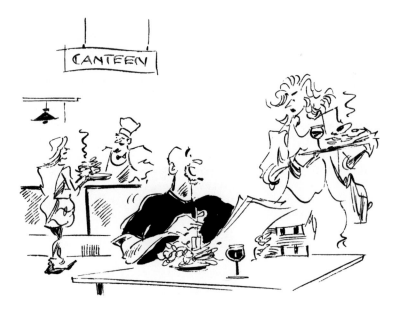

" IT'S AMAZING HOW ALL OF THE OTHER DATA SOURCES CAN BE SO WRONG. "

ADVANTAGES

✔ Naturalistic setting

✔ Allows a flexible approach to design

✔ Do-able for small-scale researcher as can be limited to one site

✔ Cost-effective method for small-scale research

DISADVANTAGES

✘ Defining the boundaries of the case can prove difficult, leading to over or under inclusion of data

✘ The findings may not easily be generalised to other settings. The transferability to other settings depends on a detailed matching of the sites rather than on statistical generalisation

References

Borckardt J 2002 Case study examining the efficacy of a multi-modal psychotherapeutic intervention for hypertension. International Journal of Clinical and Experimental Hypnosis **50**(2): 189–201

Farquhar J 1991 Objects, processes, and female infertility in Chinese medicine. Medical Anthropology Quarterly **5**(4): 370–399

Luff D, Thomas K 1999 Models of complementary therapy provision in primary care. Medical Care Research Unit School of Health and Related Research, University of Sheffield, Sheffield

Luff D, Thomas K 2000 Sustaining complementary therapy provision in primary care: lessons from existing services. Complementary Therapies in Medicine **8**(3): 173–179

Reuther I, Aldridge D 1998 Qigong Yangsheng as a complementary therapy in the management of asthma: a single-case appraisal. Journal of Alternative and Complementary Medicine **4**(2): 173–183

Yin R 1994 Case study research design and methods. Sage, Thousand Oaks, p 13

Ethnography

7

WHAT IS ETHNOGRAPHY?

Ethnography is the name used to describe an approach to research as well as the written text produced to report ethnographic research. Ethnography was developed by cultural anthropologists and sociologists to understand the behaviour and beliefs of groups of people. Ethnography is characterised by fieldwork and in that sense is an empirical approach to research. The researcher will spend an extended period of time within the culture of interest, not simply as an observer looking from a distance but as a participant observer entering into the routine as well as the organised and ritualised activities of the group. By becoming immersed in the culture, the researcher hopes to understand the insider's view of his own world. The aim is not simply to describe that world from an insider's view, but to develop a theoretical understanding of the culture. To cultivate this cultural sensitivity the ethnographer will pay attention to a wide range of cultural phenomena, including the beliefs, values, practices, relationships, rituals, language and myths of the group (Hare 1993). How these different aspects are interrelated is of central concern to the ethnographer. Attention is also given to the implicit as well as the explicit 'rules' that shape social interactions (Cowie & Roebuck 1975).

This is reported in an ethnography, which is an extended and detailed case report of the different aspects of the culture and how they are understood by the researcher. The ethnography is a form of exploratory case study in which researchers provide a detailed description and interpretation of their observations and experiences (Oths 1994). The characteristics of ethnography are given in Box 7.1.

DOING ETHNOGRAPHY

Like all forms of research, ethnography must be guided by a research question. The traditional anthropological approach to ethnography of going to a remote

---

Box 7.1   Characteristics of ethnography

- Fieldwork in which the researcher spends an extended period of time within the culture
- Participant observation through which the researcher experiences the culture first hand to gain an insider's view
- An exploratory approach towards the culture of interest rather than the testing of specific hypotheses
- Working with unstructured data largely from observations and conversations
- Focus upon one or very few cases in detail
- Analysis which attempts to explain the meaning and function of cultural phenomena 'in context'

---

culture with an open mind and no preconceptions is a useful injunction, but somewhat impractical and naive as it is impossible to be completely free from preconceptions. You should have a clear sense of why you are interested in investigating a particular culture or aspect of your own culture. The precise framing of the question may change with experience gained in the field, but without the question to guide your inquiry it is difficult to know what data you should gather.

Ethnography is used to answer questions about a culture. To study culture does not mean you have to go to exotic or faraway places (although there is an understandable appeal). Ethnography can be used to understand aspects of your own culture. Lifestyles or subgroups within a culture have been the subject of many excellent ethnographies (see Example 7.1, Cowie & Roebuck 1975, and Example 7.2, Hare 1993). You should satisfy yourself about how this study might inform the field of professional practice you are interested in.

The types of questions ethnography is suited to answering within a healthcare context include:

- **How members of a particular group perceive or understand certain social or cultural phenomena:** for example, how do mothers of young children attending a complementary medicine clinic conceive of and use vaccination?

- **How particular social or cultural practices are socially constructed among members of a certain group:** for example, how do new mothers in rural England understand the role of the health visitor?

You should think about what current theory exists for explaining the phenomenon that you are interested in and, if there is no research in this specific area, what theoretical models you will draw upon. (See section on conceptual framework in Ch. 2, General design issues.)

Example 7.1 Ethnography of a chiropractic clinic (Cowie & Roebuck 1975)

Aim

This study describes in detail the functioning of a chiropractic clinic and the marginal status held by chiropractors in 1970s America.

Strategy

Through participant observation wide-ranging data were gathered about the functioning of one chiropractic clinic. This provided a base for understanding how the identity of the chiropractor was shaped through his encounters with patients and other professionals.

Data gathering

The researcher gained access to the research site firstly as a patient and then employed as a full-time assistant to the chiropractor over a period of 14 weeks. During that time field notes, observations, conversations, interviews and documentary data were collected. The nature of the social research was not concealed from the chiropractor or his patients and there was a substantial cross-checking of the data.

Analysis

Sociological theories of deviance and marginalisation and the methods of symbolic interactionism underpinned how the study was formulated and analysed. Symbolic interactionism is a framework for unpacking the meanings given by participants to their interactions with others and the world.

In particular the concept of social deviance was used to explain the position adopted by the chiropractor in relation to his patients and other professionals.

Reporting

The ethnography took the form of a 162-page book which described in detail the researcher's own position, the theoretical framework underpinning the study, the principles of chiropractic as articulated by the chiropractor, the social and political context that surrounded the chiropractic clinic and the day-to-day functioning of the clinic. This culminated in an explanation of how the office setting was used as a stage for 'chiropractic encounters' and how these reinforced the self-identity of the chiropractor and his marginal status in American society.

Negotiating access

Having decided upon your topic area, you will need to negotiate access to the group you are interested in. There are a number of issues you will need to consider. The first is how open you will be regarding your role as a researcher.

Example 7.2   Ethnography: the emergence of an urban US Chinese medicine (Hare 1993)

Aim
To describe how Chinese medicine principles and practice are incorporated in an urban US setting.

Strategy
Through participant observation to understand how users and practitioners of Chinese medicine utilise the theories of Chinese medicine to address twentieth century US urban concerns.

Data gathering
Between 1998 and 2000 the researcher became a participant observer attending two municipally run acupuncture detoxification clinics for drug and alcohol addiction. Access was also gained to five practising acupuncturists (Chinese immigrant as well as US trained) who invited the researcher to 'hang out', observe their work and talk to their patients.

The sampling strategy was opportunistic and took advantage of 'snowballing' (see Ch. 11, Sampling). Through the above activities plus attending meetings, seminars and social events, a sample of 30 practitioners and 29 patients was developed. The patients were all non-Asian, predominantly middle income, except for the detox patients who tended to be lower income.

Analysis
The conceptual framework for the analysis was based on Kleinman's theory of explanatory models (Kleinman 1980). An explanatory model is any attempt to understand illness and treatment. This is based on the dichotomy between disease (physician's domain) and illness (patient's domain).

Confucian theories of order and moderation as well as a late twentieth century belief in individual responsibility for health were brought together in relation to how a person can maintain or restore health.

The analytic process, while not described in great detail, focused upon how the discourse of patients and practitioners can be constructed to show a new synthesis of US urban oriental medicine.

Reporting
The ethnography was reported in a 19-page journal article. A brief background and methods section was followed by the analysis of patients' and practitioners' models of health and illness and how their language revealed an emerging synthesis of traditional Confucian concepts of order and moderation and US individualism.

The purpose of participant observation is to gather your data in a naturalistic setting to get an insider's view. If everyone in the group you are studying is aware of you as a researcher, their behaviour and the conversations you have may be significantly affected by this fact. This potential limitation must be balanced with the ethical demand to gain informed consent. The principle of informed consent is a widely accepted ethical requirement for engaging others in your research. (See section on informed consent in Ch. 4, Research ethics.)

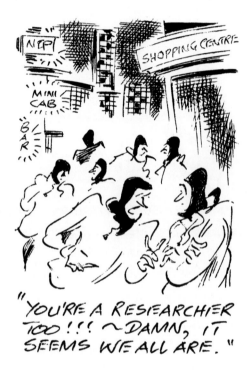

Gaining access is dependent upon your having sufficient personal credentials to enter the group, whether those be age, colour, gender or other markers of social groups such as particular skills or talents. An ethnography of traditional Islamic women's beliefs about gender relationships could really only be done by a woman with access to that culture. Everyone is excluded from certain social groups on the basis of personal characteristics, and gaining initial access and sufficient trust is dependent upon our having the requisite credentials.

You will probably need to negotiate access to your site of research with formal and/or informal gatekeepers. These are people who hold positions of authority within the group you are interested in, and gaining access to the site may be dependent upon their permission. Your relationships with these people may be important for gaining access to a site but also as a basis for building trust with the group you are interested in. It takes more than the granting of permission to be trusted with 'insider knowledge', and the first step in building sufficient trust starts with the gatekeepers who are the initial guarantors of your credibility as a researcher. Rather than being a one-off event, negotiating access is a continual process throughout the period of your involvement with the site.

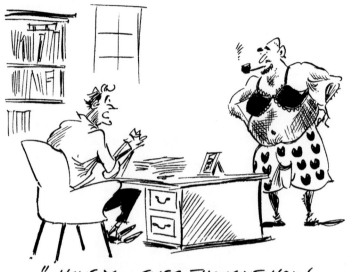

" HAVE YOU EVER THOUGHT HOW BETRAYED THESE WOMEN WILL FEEL IF, SOMEHOW, THEY DISCOVER YOU'RE A MAN? "

Data collection

PARTICIPATION AND OBSERVATION

The basis of data collection is your participation in and observation of the culture you are studying. There are varying degrees of participation and observation and you should think about how you wish to position yourself in the group:

- How fully you are able to participate in the range of the group's activities will influence your own insights as well as how you are seen by other members within the group.
- How far you consciously choose to adopt the orientation of an insider will influence your understanding of the phenomenon.
- Who within the group knows about your role as a researcher and what they know about the research may influence the quality of your interactions and the data you are able to collect.

FIELD NOTES

It is important to keep detailed records of the events you observe, conversations you might have and your own perceptions. You may not think so at the time, but it is all too easy to forget many of the details unless they are written down very soon after the event. The sorts of things you should record in all your fieldnotes include:

- The time, date and place of the observations
- Specific facts, numbers, details of what happens at the site
- Sensory impressions, i.e. sights, sounds, textures, smells, tastes
- Specific words, phrases, summaries of conversations, and insider language
- Your own response to the events
- Questions for further investigation.

INTERVIEWS

In addition to your role as a participant observer you will probably want to conduct interviews. These range from informal conversations as you participate in activities to more formal interviews, with the aim of finding out more about specific aspects of the culture. Interviews provide a chance to learn how people reflect directly on behaviour, circumstances, identity, events and other things. This information will help you understand the insider's view, which is central for ethnography. If you decide to conduct a formal interview you should try to be clear about what you want to find out from the interview. Explore the area of interest with open-ended questions, but if respondents head off on a tangent don't be too quick to have them return to your prepared agenda. These deviations may lead to useful information that you did not know was needed.

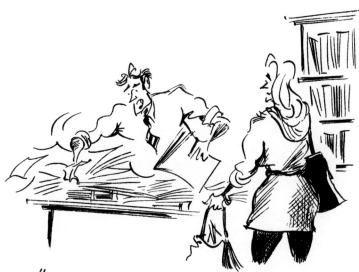

" HMM, YOU'VE MADE A VERY
INTERESTING POINT ~ I'LL SEE
IF I CAN FIND A QUESTION
TO GO WITH IT. "

Where possible, make tape recordings of your formal interviews (be sure to get explicit permission for this from the person you are interviewing). At the very least make detailed notes, as described above for field notes. (See Ch. 12 Interviews, and Ch. 14, Observations.)

Data analysis

The first step in the creation of an ethnography is to provide detailed descriptions of the site being studied. This may be in terms of the physical characteristics, the people involved, specific events and happenings. Your own interpretation of how these different aspects are linked is the foundation of your analysis (try to see it in the light of your guiding research question and your conceptual framework). This process of description and interpretation begins early on in the project, and as your ideas are refined further questions will be raised. You will then try to answer these questions with further fieldwork. In this way the analysis is built up as you develop different lines of inquiry to answer your research questions. Further detail on this will be found in Chapter 16, Analysing qualitative data.

REFLEXIVITY

Within the ethnographic tradition it is well understood that the presentation of research findings is not simply a question of describing things from a truly objective position, but of the researcher's own interpretation of the events. How you describe and make sense of the events you observe will be based on your own cultural and social background as well as on personal experiences. Because the researcher's own interpretation is central to ethnography, it is important to be explicit about how your own beliefs and background influence what you see. This is known as reflexivity. You should include sufficient detail about your own background, and about professional and personal experiences that might have a bearing on the way you have interpreted the data. Whilst you will want to provide just enough information so that the reader is in a position to evaluate these influences, you should ensure that your ethnography does not turn into an autobiography — another research method altogether. It is usual to provide some form of introduction in a preface or introductory section of a report, explaining the personal relevance of the topic to the researcher, and something of the experience or perspectives the researcher has brought to the study, but reflexivity does not stop there. Throughout the text it may be appropriate for researchers to make reference to the way their background and perspectives have influenced what has been seen and how that information was analysed.

 Because the researcher's own interpretation is central to ethnography, it is important to be explicit about how your own beliefs and background influence what you see.

THEORETICAL DEVELOPMENT

Because you are going beyond a description of events into interpretation, you will need to be explicit about the theories you have used to make sense of your observations and experience. The theories may come from your professional training, from personal experience or from the literature. Making these known helps the reader understand where you are coming from and how you have put the pieces together. The theories you use will help generate the questions that guide your research and link your work to broader questions about cultural processes and how they come into play within your particular setting. This link to the broader context is important because your description and interpretation become part of a wider field of research. You should give consideration to how your findings tie in with or contradict what others have found.

Whilst there is no single overarching theory that is correct for making sense of all social and cultural processes, there are a variety of theoretical models that have been used to understand culture. Theories about the socially constructed nature of gender roles is an example of this (Goldberger et al 1987). Gender as an analytic concept might help you make sense of the way different social groups divide responsibilities and assets, develop social and kinship relationships and many other aspects of men's and women's lives (Farquhar 1991).

Other theories focus on the use of symbols in human interaction. Within this framework symbols are thought to convey cultural meaning, and how symbols are interpreted within a culture provides insight into the beliefs and values held by that culture (Cowie & Roebuck 1975). There are numerous other theories that can inform your analysis, from the exercise of power (Foucault 1970) to post-modern deconstructionism (Derrida 1982). The theories you call on will depend upon your research focus and the questions you are trying to answer. Whichever theories you use to develop your interpretation, try and be explicit about how and when you are using them (Denzin 1997). (See the section on conceptual frameworks in Ch. 2, General design issues.)

VALIDITY

The validity of an ethnography is based upon a number of factors. The first is that the researcher spends an extended period of time in the research setting, for professional researchers this may be months to years. Through a prolonged engagement and drawing on all their perceptions and experiences, the researcher interprets events with a sensitivity for the insider's view. The researcher provides sufficient 'thick description' of the context in which events occur to enable the reader to evaluate the evidence for the theoretical links that the researcher proposes. Researchers make no pretence at being a photographic plate that records objectively what happens within the research setting, rather they are obliged to declare significant factors such as background, professional and personal experience, theoretical interests and the research focus that shapes their view. Going further than simply stating that these influences exist, the researcher needs to show how and where these influences have informed the analysis.

ADVANTAGES

✔ Provides an in-depth holistic account which is rich in contextual detail

✔ Based on first-hand observation and experience

✔ Is able to presents the insider's viewpoint

✔ Can be used to develop and extend the theoretical understanding of a culture or sub-culture

✔ Does not attempt to exclude the researcher's own experience and perceptions

✔ Through reflexivity the researcher's potential to influence data collection and theory development is acknowledged

DISADVANTAGES

✘ Requires an extended period of involvement with the site which may not fit with the demands for completing the research within a limited time frame

✘ Gaining access to research sites may prove problematic

✘ The researcher's presence may disturb the naturalness of the situation, thereby jeopardising the whole purpose of the ethnographic approach — seeing things in their natural context

✘ Demands the researcher maintains a high level of self-awareness — reflexivity

References

Cowie J, Roebuck J 1975 An ethnography of a chiropractic clinic. The Free Press, Macmillan, New York

Denzin N 1997 Interpretive ethnography: ethnographic practices for the 21st century. Sage, Thousand Oak

Derrida J 1982 Margins of philosophy. (Trans. Bass A) University of Chicago Press, Chicago

Farquhar J 1991 Objects, processes, and female infertility in Chinese medicine. Medical Anthropology Quarterly 5(4): 370–399

Foucault M 1970 The order of things: an archaeology of the human sciences. Vintage, New York

Goldberger N, Clinchy B et al 1987 Women's ways of knowing: on gaining a voice. In: Shaver P, Hendrick C (eds) Sex and gender. SPHC, Sage, Newbury Park, p 201–228

Hare M 1993 The emergence of an urban US Chinese medicine. Medical Anthropology Quarterly 7(1): 30–49

Kleinman A 1980 Patients and healers in the context of culture: an exploration of the borderland between anthropology, medicine, and psychiatry. University of California Press, Berkeley

Oths K 1994 Communication in a chiropractic clinic: how a DC treats his patients. Culture, Medicine and Psychiatry 18(1): 83–113

Further reading

Chiseri-Strater E, Stone Sunstein B 1997 Fieldworking: reading and writing research. Blair Press, Upper Saddle River, NJ, p 73

Spradley JP 1980 Participant observation. Holt, Rinehart and Winston, New York

Taylor S (ed) 2002 Ethnographic research: a reader. Sage, London

Experiments and quasi-experiments

8

INTRODUCTION

The term experimental research conjures up images of labs, white coats and technical apparatus to measure the effects of the experiment, but there is much more to experimental research than this. Sure enough, a lot of experiments do take place in the lab, but one of the most important research tools used in health care to evaluate the effects of treatment is the clinical trial — a classic example of a field experiment. Although conducting a clinical trial is beyond the scope of most students or independent practitioners, the principles of experimental design are important to understand.

The basis of an experiment is pretty straightforward, i.e. to observe the effects of an intervention. We all conduct experiments in our daily lives. Yesterday we cooked pasta for 8 minutes and it was a bit too chewy so today we try a bit more, say 10 minutes. We observe, or in the case of the pasta feel and taste, the results — softer pasta — 'al dente' with any luck. If we try a different route from home to work or university to see if it is quicker, easier or cheaper we are engaging in an experiment of daily living. The difference between these experiments and the kind that would pass muster as research is having a clearly stated hypothesis and the degree of attention given to factors that might confound the results. Experiments can be used to isolate individual factors and observe their effects in detail, such as the effectiveness of a particular treatment. They can also be used to discover new relationships or properties and to put theories to the test.

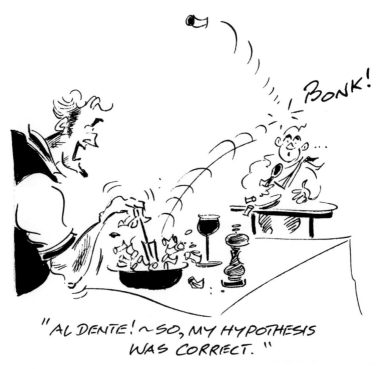

"AL DENTE! ~ SO, MY HYPOTHESIS WAS CORRECT."

MANIPULATION

Experimental methods took a kick-start during the scientific revolution, with investigators wanting to increase the precision and accuracy of their research and to decrease the influence of confounding factors. No longer satisfied to rely on the opinions of the great writers from the past, they began to engage in direct observation and experimentation. While the most dramatic developments were in the laboratory with its controlled conditions — ideal for chemistry and physics — the last 50 years have seen the methods rigorously applied in clinical conditions in real human beings. Whether it is in the lab or in the field, the requirements for an experiment are that the researcher is able to control and actively manipulate an intervention, and reliably record the outcome. The observations and measurements need to be precise and detailed so the researcher can say with confidence that the intervention has a positive, negative or zero effect on the condition. In the jargon the intervention is called the *independent variable* and the condition that the intervention is designed to influence is the *dependent variable*. The independent variable is manipulated and the effect is observed on the dependent variable. It is crucial that the researcher is able to pre-specify what the key variables are. To stick with our pasta example, the softness of the pasta is the dependent variable that we want to influence, and the cooking time is the independent variable that we are using. We need to be confident that it is cooking time and not temperature, altitude or water to pasta ratio that is the crucial independent variable. In this respect an experimental strategy differs from a case study or action research, where precise areas of influence may not be clearly identified at the outset of the research.

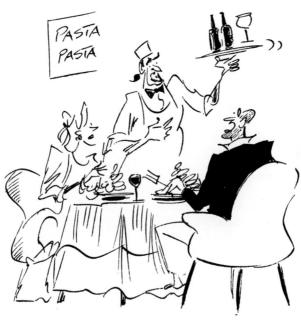

"TELL CHEF TO SORT OUT
HIS INDEPENDENT VARIABLE."

Control of confounding factors

Researchers need to be able to control the intervention and circumstances surrounding their experiments to ensure that results are not being influenced by other interfering variables. The laboratory is the ultimate in control and it is for this reason that some research is conducted exclusively in these controlled conditions, but real life is not hermetically sealed, and what holds in the lab can be different in the real world where the results are to be used. Field researchers have to find other ways of meeting this challenge. They may be able to control some variables such as where and when the intervention is given; however, it is not possible to control all the variables that may affect the results of the study. That is why control groups are used.

CONTROL GROUPS

The control group is matched to the intervention group in important characteristics, for example age, sex, chronicity of condition etc., but the control group do not receive the independent variable (the intervention). At the end of the study the dependent variable (the condition) is measured and if the two groups differ then the researcher can surmise that it was due to the independent variable (the intervention). If the experiment is evaluating a treatment, then withholding all treatment from a control group might be unethical if the standard treatment was accepted to be of value. One way of addressing this ethical concern is to have the control group receive the standard treatment and the experimental group receive the new treatment. This is viable when the standard treatment has been conclusively shown to be of benefit. It then acts as a benchmark. If the standard treatment is unproven, then it remains unclear what, if any, benefit either the standard or the experimental treatment is having above and beyond no treatment. This is an important consideration in those conditions that tend to resolve naturally over time without any treatment, such as the common cold, muscle strain etc.

SAMPLING

When it is impossible or impractical to work with the entire population, sampling is used to choose a subset of the population. In experimental designs where the aim is to create findings that can be generalised to the wider population, some form of probability sampling is used. This is so that the experimental group is representative of the wider population in terms of defined characteristics. A range of techniques for achieving this are explained in Chapter 11, Sampling, but the most commonly used is randomisation.

RANDOMISATION

Random selection is designed to reduce the risk of systematic bias by ensuring that those included in the sample are representative of the population from which they were drawn. *Random assignment* is where those in the selected sample are given an equal chance of being assigned into either the treatment group or the control group. This straightforward randomisation into the two 'arms' of the study works well when the population is fairly homogeneous and the sample is large. If the sample included in each arm does not have sufficient numbers to be a fair representation of a diverse group, then this can bias the results through the exclusion of minorities. This can be corrected by stratifying the sample. Chapter 11, Sampling, explains this in greater detail.

Outcome measures

The choice of outcome measure will depend upon the dependent variable being measured. If the variable of interest is a change in blood chemistry, then specific blood tests related to that variable will be required. On the other hand, if a particular symptom such as low back pain is the variable of interest, then a self-report questionnaire may be the outcome measure of choice. An observation schedule or self-report questionnaire may be appropriate if the dependent variable is a change of behaviour. For general wellbeing and specific diseases there is a wide range of established outcome measures such as the SF–36 discussed below (in Example 8.3, p 92–93) (Bowling 1991, 1995).

Established outcome measures have generally gone through various stages of testing for their validity and reliability. It is important that the instrument is able to evaluate effectively the essential elements related to the condition being studied. If a back pain measure fails to include important elements such as mobility, effect on sleep or use of analgesia, then the validity of the measure will be called into question. It is also important that the instrument is sufficiently sensitive to modest degrees of change in the condition. If a test is repeated (within a brief time frame) and the scores are not comparable then its (test–retest) reliability is called into question.

The *Chiropractic Revised Oswestry Pain Questionnaire* (Fig. 8.1) is a widely used outcome measure in back pain research. It has 10 sections, each addressing a different aspect of back pain. The question asked in each section has a series of six graded responses scored from 0–5 for which a single answer may be given. The overall score is then totalled to a maximum of 50.

A review of the clinical research literature should provide information on the measures that have been used and that appear to be generally acceptable. For many diseases, however, relevant measures are still being defined. In addition, evaluating a holistic treatment approach may require new patient-related outcomes measures (Long et al 2000). In response to an increased focus on the patient's experience of health interventions, patient-generated outcome measures have been developed.

One that has been employed in several studies of complementary therapies is known as MYMOP (Measure Yourself Medical Outcome Profile) (Paterson 1996), shown in Figure 8.2. At the first consultation the patient chooses one or two symptoms, and one activity of daily living which he or she considers the most important. The items must all relate, in the patient's opinion, to the same problem. These choices are written down in the patient's own words and are then scored on a seven-point scale. The patient also scores general wellbeing. At the next follow-up the wording of the previously chosen items remains unchanged but there is an optional fifth item for a new symptom. Follow-up questionnaires can be administered postally or during subsequent consultations.

EXPERIMENTAL DESIGNS

There are several variations in how and when an intervention is evaluated. These are described below.

THE CHIROPRACTIC REVISED OSWESTRY PAIN QUESTIONNAIRE

Name _____   Today's Date: _____

Please read carefully: This questionnaire is designed to enable us to understand how much your low back pain has affected your ability to manage your everyday activities. Please circle the LETTER that most closely describes your situation.

1   Pain Intensity

- The pain comes and goes and is very mild.
- The pain is mild and does not vary much.
- The pain comes and goes and is moderate.
- The pain is moderate and does not vary much.
- The pain comes and goes and is severe.
- The pain is severe and does not vary much.

2   Personal Care

- I do not have to change my way of washing or dressing in order to avoid pain.
- I do not normally change my way of washing or dressing even though it causes some pain.
- Washing and dressing increase the pain, but I manage not to change my way of doing it.
- Washing and dressing increase the pain and I find it necessary to change my way of doing it.
- Because of the pain, I am unable to do some washing and dressing without help.
- Because of the pain, I am unable to do any washing or dressing without help.

3   Lifting

- I can lift heavy weights without extra pain.
- I can lift heavy weights but it gives me extra pain.
- Pain prevents me from lifting heavy weights off the floor.
- Pain prevents me from lifting heavy weights off the floor, but I can manage if they are conveniently positioned, e.g. on a table.
- Pain prevents me from lifting heavy weights, but I can manage light to medium weights if they are conveniently positioned.
- I can only lift very light weights, at the most.

4   Walking

- I have no pain on walking.
- I have some pain with walking but it does not increase with distance.
- I cannot walk more than 1 mile without increasing pain.
- I cannot walk more than 1/2 mile without increasing pain.
- I cannot walk more than 1/4 mile without increasing pain.
- I cannot walk at all without increasing pain.

5   Sitting

- I can sit in any chair as long as I like.
- I can only sit in my favourite chair as long as I like.
- Pain prevents me sitting for more than 1 hour.
- Pain prevents me sitting for more than 1/2 hour.
- Pain prevents me sitting for more than 10 minutes.
- I avoid sitting because it increases pain straight away.

6   Standing

- I can stand as long as I want without pain.
- I have some pain while standing, but it does not increase with time.

- I cannot stand for longer than 1 hour without increasing pain.
- I cannot stand for longer than 1/2 hour without increasing pain.
- I cannot stand for longer than 10 minutes without increasing pain.
- I avoid standing because it increases pain straight away.

7 Sleeping

- I get no pain in bed.
- I get pain in bed, but it does not prevent me from sleeping well.
- Because of pain, my normal night's sleep is reduced by less than one-quarter.
- Because of pain, my normal night's sleep is reduced by less than one-half.
- Because of pain, my normal night's sleep is reduced by less than three-quarters.
- Pain prevents me from sleeping at all.

8 Social Life

- My social life is normal and gives me no pain.
- My social life is normal, but increases the degree of my pain.
- Pain has no significant effect on my social life apart from limiting my more energetic interests, e.g. dancing, etc.
- Pain has restricted my social life and I do not go out very often.

- Pain has restricted my social life to my home.
- I have hardly any social life because of the pain.

9 Travelling

- I get no pain while travelling.
- I get some pain while travelling, but none of my usual forms of travel make it any worse.
- I get extra pain while travelling, but it does not compel me to seek alternative forms of travel.
- I get extra pain while travelling which compels me to seek alternative forms of travel.
- Pain restricts all forms of travel.
- Pain prevents all forms of travel except that done lying down.

10 Changing Degree of Pain

- My pain is rapidly getting better.
- My pain fluctuates, but overall is definitely getting better.
- My pain seems to be getting better, but improvement is slow at present.
- My pain is neither getting better nor worse.
- My pain is gradually worsening.
- My pain is rapidly worsening.

Examiner:_____

Figure 8.1 The Chiropractic revised Oswestry pain questionnaire (from the Oswestry website www.merc.wlv.ac.uk, with permission of the authors).

The classic design

This begins with random selection of the sample followed by random assignment into two groups. The dependent variable is then measured (pre-test) in both groups — those who will receive the intervention and those who will not receive the intervention. At this point the researcher can check to see the two groups are comparable and have similar scores. This is an important consideration especially when samples are small. The next stage is the introduction of the intervention to the first group. The dependent variable is then measured again (post-test) in both groups. If the intervention had no effect then the scores of both groups should be similar. If you want to check whether the effects of the intervention are enduring then a *follow-up evaluation* of the dependent variable can be put in place.

MYMOP2 Follow up

Full name ....   Today's date ....

Please circle the number to show how severe your problem has been IN THE LAST WEEK. This should be YOUR opinion, no-one else's!

SYMPTOM 1:   0   1   2   3   4   5   6
....   As good as   As bad as
....   it could be   it could be

SYMPTOM 2:   0   1   2   3   4   5   6
....   As good as   As bad as
....   it could be   it could be

ACTIVITY: 0   1   2   3   4   5   6
....   As good as   As bad as
....   it could be   it could be

WELLBEING: 0   1   2   3   4   5   6
How would you   As good as   As bad as
rate your   it could be   it could be
general feeling
of wellbeing?

If an important new symptom has appeared please describe it and mark how bad it is below. Otherwise do not use this line.

SYMPTOM 3:   0   1   2   3   4   5   6
....   As good as   As bad as
....   it could be   it could be

The treatment you are receiving may not be the only thing affecting your problem. If there is anything else that you think is important, such as changes you have made yourself, or other things happening in your life, please write it here (write overleaf if you need more space):

Are you taking medication FOR THIS PROBLEM ? Please circle: YES/NO
IF YES:
Please write in name of medication, and how much a day/week

....
....

MYMOP, Measure Yourself Medical Outcome Profile

For instructions for use and to check for up-to-date version and information, please visit website http://www.hsrc.ac.uk/mymop or contact Dr Charlotte Paterson at C. Paterson@bristol.ac.uk

Figure 8.2 The MYMOP questionnaire. (From Paterson C 1996 Measuring outcomes in primary care: a patient generated measure, MYMOP, compared with the SF–36 health survey. British Medical Journal 312: 1016–1020.)

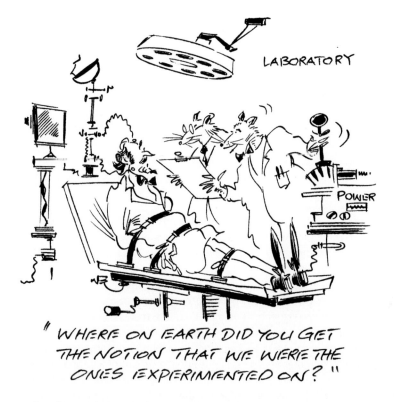

LABORATORY

POWER

" WHERE ON EARTH DID YOU GET
THE NOTION THAT WE WERE THE
ONES EXPERIMENTED ON? "

Another variation is the *crossover trial* in which the group receiving the intervention is alternated. In effect, the participants become their own control. This principle is discussed further in relation to N=1 single case studies on page 88 (Hansen & Hansen 1983).

Factorial design

The simple approach to experimentation described above can be developed by having multiple dependent and independent variables. A subgroup might be identified who have had the condition being studied (the dependent variable) over a longer period of time than the rest. Another possibility is that the dosage of the independent variable is altered for a subgroup. Each new variable adds a complexity to the design and increases the number of participants required so that each category has sufficient participants for meaningful analysis. The statistics required to interpret the results also become more complex. Whilst being able to measure a range of variables in one study may seem attractive, if there are insufficient data collected due to poor recruitment, drop out or incorrect data entry, then establishing statistical significance may not be possible. It is advisable to seek the help of a statistician at design stage to ensure that there is sufficient statistical power to evaluate whether the changes are due to more than chance factors. This will depend upon the degree of change predicted between the intervention and non-intervention groups as well as the numbers in each sub-sample. See the section on statistics in Chapter 17, Analysing quantitative data, for further explanation.

Post-test only design

It is sometimes advocated that in certain instances one can omit the pre-test phase of the research. If the intervention is teaching motor skills, and the pre-test evaluates those same skills then taking that test becomes part of the learning. The difficulty with this approach is that without the pre-test we do not have a baseline upon which we could evaluate any change or know whether the two groups differed prior to the intervention. Randomisation goes some way to addressing the potential for difference between groups, but does not allow us to confidently infer if there has been any change.

Pre-test post-test without controls

Although uncontrolled studies might not provide the strongest evidence of effectiveness, they can be a useful first stage in the development of more rigorous studies. They can provide some evidence of the effects of an intervention (White & Ernst 2001). The single group is tested before and after the intervention. Without a control group there is no reference point for judging the effectiveness of an intervention, unless it can be benchmarked against other research. It is also difficult to make comparisons with other research unless you can be sure that you are comparing like with like. With conditions that tend to improve spontaneously over time, the lack of a control group means that it is not possible to judge whether the intervention has made a difference. If it is not feasible to have a control group, then a case study approach should be considered, where a range of data sources and collection methods can support the validity of the findings. With case study the focus is not upon simple cause and effect but on contextualising the findings.

Solomon four group design

This method overcomes the disadvantages of pre-test interference by having four groups:

- Group 1 receives the pre-test, then the intervention, followed by a post-test
- Group 2 receives the pre-test and post-test but no intervention
- Group 3 receives no pre-test but the intervention and post-test are given
- Group 4 only the post-test is given.

By comparing the post-test results the researcher is able to evaluate the effect of the intervention by comparing the experimental (1 and 3) and control (2 and 4) groups. In addition, by comparing groups 1 and 3 and groups 2 and 4 the researcher can detect any interaction between the pre-test and the intervention. Whilst this is a powerful research design, the necessity for a large sample to randomise into four groups and the time taken in organisation and analysis of the experiment makes it unrealistic for most small-scale researchers working with a human population.

EXPERIMENTING IN THE REAL WORLD

The randomised controlled trial

Whilst a full-scale randomised controlled trial (RCT) is beyond the scope of students or solo practitioner researchers, it is important to understand it as an exemplar of field experiments. A good RCT will conform to the principles described above for experiments in terms of manipulation of variables, the control of confounding factors and, of course, sampling and randomisation. The well-designed and -conducted RCT has become the gold standard for evaluating treatment efficacy in health research. This is achieved by utilising an array of stringent safeguards and checks against potential confounding factors and bias.

The RCT is not the only way of evaluating interventions and its use is sometimes impossible or unethical but, when it is relevant and well conducted, it provides the most reliable evidence of efficacy.

There are different kinds of RCTs. An *explanatory* or *fastidious RCT* maintains a high degree of control over the dependent and independent variables, ensuring that the only significant difference between the two groups is the specific intervention. Take for example the trial by Reilly et al (1986) which tested the hypothesis that homeopathic potencies are not active. In this carefully conducted study the only identifiable difference between the two groups was that one group were given a placebo medicine and the other group were given the homeopathic medicine. The results showed that those in the group receiving the homeopathy had fewer symptoms of hayfever and used fewer antihistamines than those in the placebo group.

A *pragmatic RCT* evaluates treatments as they are delivered in the real world. The low back pain study by Meade et al (1990) comparing chiropractic and standard outpatient hospital treatment is a good example of a pragmatic trial. In this case both groups received the treatment normally offered at a chiropractic clinic or an outpatients' department. The comparison was not of manipulation or any specific aspect of the treatment. Rather, the comparison was between the two packages as a whole. The practitioners were at liberty to adjust the treatment regimes as they saw fit for individual patients and to give the number of treatments they thought were necessary. The differences reflected the usual policy for treatment of mechanical low back pain. The advantage of the pragmatic approach is that it compares treatments as they are given in day-to-day practice without pre-specifying what manoeuvre or how many treatments are to be given to a particular patient. The disadvantage of the pragmatic approach is that it is impossible to identify the precise components of the intervention that are responsible for the observed difference. This is sometimes less important than knowing that a particular therapeutic approach is the most effective strategy for a particular problem – whatever the precise mechanisms of action (Cardini & Weixin 1998).

N=1

Also known as a single subject (or case) experimental design or a time series study, an N=1 is essentially an experiment where the case acts as its own control. Once a baseline (A) is established of the important (dependent) variable in the case (for instance blood pressure), an intervention (say a herb) is introduced and the dependent variables (B) are measured. The intervention is then stopped and following a 'wash out' period the dependent variables are again measured (A). The process can be repeated and is sometimes referred to as an ABAB design (see Fig. 8.3a). This cycle of *testing–intervention–testing–non-intervention–testing* can be reiterated and in this way the single case becomes its own control.

A basic requirement for making the case act as its own control is a stable baseline. In individual health terms this would mean a chronic stable condition rather than an acute or self-limiting illness. A second requirement is that the effects of the intervention do not persist once the intervention is stopped. This is to be sure that the non-intervention phase measurements are not picking up on the carry-over effects of the intervention. Variations on this design include adding a new intervention, an ABAC design (see Fig. 8. 3a). A is the baseline of the dependent variable, such as a sign or symptom; B is the intervention, the second A is measurement of the dependent variable after a wash out period; and C is the introduction of a new intervention.

It is also possible to set multiple baselines for measurement. Rather than relying on a single baseline like blood pressure, a range of baselines relevant to the investigation are included, such as signs, symptoms or scoring of outcome measures.

The crucial factor determining suitability for this strategy, where there is an alternation between intervention and non-intervention stages, is that the effects of the intervention are not long lasting. If the effects carry on through the non-intervention phase, then this will obscure the non-intervention response. Pain relief interventions where the pain is chronic and fairly stable

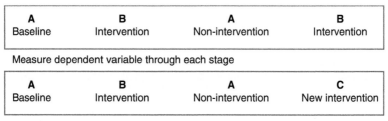

A Baseline	**B** Intervention	**A** Non-intervention	**B** Intervention

Measure dependent variable through each stage

A Baseline	**B** Intervention	**A** Non-intervention	**C** New intervention

Figure 8.3a   N=1 design.

could be studied with this approach (Vincent 1990) (see Example 8.1). The example by Reuther and Aldridge (1998) assumes that their intervention does have persistent effects and their design does not alternate between baseline A and intervention B (see Fig. 8.3b in Example 8.2). Their variation on the N=1 design alternates between different aspects of the intervention and then compares the follow-up with the original baseline.

Example 8.1   Single group time series (Vincent 1990)

A single case design, with time series analysis, was employed to evaluate the efficacy of acupuncture in the treatment of tension headache. Fourteen patients were given eight weekly treatments, four of true acupuncture and four of sham in random order. Mean pain in medication scores were reduced by 52% and 54% respectively at initial follow-up. Reductions in pain scores of over 50% were achieved by half the patients and the significance of these changes confirmed by time series analysis. The majority of patients maintained their gains at 4-month follow-up. True acupuncture was shown to be significantly superior to sham, demonstrating a specific therapeutic action, in four patients. In the remainder no difference was observed.

QUASI-EXPERIMENTAL DESIGNS

This is where an experimental intervention is used but there is no random assignment to a treatment and control group. There are numerous variants on this theme and some have major shortcomings, but there are times when practical or ethical considerations require modification of the more rigorous randomised controlled trial. Rather than describing a set of strictly defined designs, quasi-experimentation implies a flexibility to adapt the concept of the experiment to real-world demands. While they may not be able to establish causation or efficacy with as much certainty as the randomised controlled experiment, when quasi-experiments are used with an awareness of their limitations they are useful tools for the real-world researcher. Researchers have to accept that they will not be able to have control over all the variables as they might in a laboratory, but they will be able to study the results of an intervention in its real-world setting (see Example 8.3, Richardson 1995, 2001a, 2001b).

Observational studies

MATCHED CONTROL STUDIES

In these studies the variable of interest is something beyond the control of the researcher. These observational studies are sometimes described as *natural experiments*. They may be natural in the sense of a spontaneously occurring event or an intervention introduced for purposes other than the research. This could be

Example 8.2   N=1 Qigong for asthma (Reuther & Aldridge 1998)

Reuther and Aldridge (1998) conducted a pilot study into the usefulness of Qigong — a breathing, movement and mental exercise — as a complementary therapeutic measure for chronic bronchial asthma.

Aim
The aim was to establish whether Qigong exercises would be a useful complementary treatment in chronic bronchial asthma.

Objectives
- Recruit study participants: through a self-referral process asthma sufferers of varying degrees of severity were integrated into existing Qigong classes run by the Family Education Institute in Bonn.
- Evaluate the changes: in peak expiratory flow (PEF) measurements, medication usage and self-report symptoms over 52 weeks, during which the self-help technique was taught.

Design
A single case series design was used as a pilot for a randomised controlled trial. Thirty individuals completed the study. There was no mention in the paper of the drop-out rate or the total population who were eligible to join the study.

Multiple variables were evaluated: peak expiratory flow (PEF), medication usage, exercise levels and self-report symptoms.

The study was divided into a number of stages:

- A   in the first stage baseline data on each individual were collected
- B   participants joined a regular class of Qigong for 8 weeks
- C   self-practice of Qigong without instruction was continued
- B2 participants joined a Qigong refresher course for 4 weeks (throughout the above phases daily peak flow and diary recordings were made)
- C2 participants continued self-practice of Qigong for 6 months without further instruction

← Daily peak flow and diary recording →					
A Baseline data	**B** Qigong course	**C** Self practice	**B2** Qigong refresher course	**C2** Self practice	**A2** Peak flow and diary follow-up
4 weeks	8 weeks	8 weeks	4 weeks	6 months	4 weeks

Figure 8.3b   Research design studies.

- **A2** 4 week follow-up period during which participants made peak flow and diary recordings. The follow-up period was a year after the initial baseline data were collected, to account for the seasonal fluctuations in asthma. The baseline data A and the follow-up data A2 were gathered in the same season (see Fig. 8.3b).

Outcome measures

Multiple variables were evaluated including peak expiratory flow (PEF), medication usage, exercise levels and structured subjective reporting of symptom changes recorded in a diary. The symptoms included sleeping through the night, dyspnoea, coughing, expectoration and general wellbeing. Secondary measures of emergency medical consultations, hospitalisation rate, antibiotic use and days off work due to asthma were compared with the year prior to the study.

Results

Each case was evaluated against its own baseline. The results are of individuals rather than average scores of the whole sample. Examples were reported in the paper.

Identifiable differences in PEF variability were found between those who continued with the exercise and those who did no more than attend the course of instruction. This indicates that adherence to the self-help regime is a crucial component.

There were cost savings across the group in terms of the secondary measures such as days off work, emergency consultations and hospitalisation and antibiotic usage.

a healthcare intervention, a behaviour such as smoking, or the workstation set up in an office. If the researcher wanted to study the impact of bereavement on immune response it would clearly be both impractical and unethical to use a controlled experiment. What is needed is a comparison group who are matched across a range of categories except the one being studied — in this case bereavement. By analysing the differences in immune response between the groups, the researcher attempts to identify whether exposure to the independent variable is a risk factor or is causative of the outcome or effect being studied.

A key weakness of using a matched control group is that the similarity between the groups may be less than that achieved by randomisation. There is the risk that any difference shown between the groups is an artefact of the recruiting method rather than the variable being studied (see Example 8.4, Bagnel et al 1990).

RETROSPECTIVE STUDIES

A retrospective study attempts to establish relationships between some event or occurrence in the past and a current state. In this type of study, sometimes described as *ex post facto* or 'after the fact', the crucial variables cannot be

Example 8.3   Quasi-experiment (Richardson 1995, 2001a, 2001b)

Richardson's evaluation study lent itself to a quasi-experimental design as a natural control group was generated by waiting lists.

Aim

To investigate the health status effects on patients referred to a complementary therapy service (osteopathy, acupuncture and homeopathy) offered within an NHS trust. It was hypothesised that there would be a difference in the health status between those receiving the treatment and those in the control group.

Design

The choice of a quasi-experimental design was pragmatic in that the number of referrals to the service far exceeded the provision allowed for by initial funding. This led to the establishment of a waiting list. Those who were first referred to the service entered the treatment arm of the study while those who were referred later had to be placed on a waiting list – they became the control group.

Outcome (SF–36)

A baseline and outcome assessment of all participants was taken using the SF–36, a general wellbeing questionnaire evaluating eight health concepts. These eight concepts are divided into:
- physical functioning
- role limitation due to physical health problems
- bodily pain
- social functioning
- psychological distress and wellbeing
- role limitation due to emotional problems
- energy levels
- general health perceptions.

The eight concepts are divided into 36 questions measured on a linear scale with a minimum total score of 0 (poor health) to a maximum of 100 (best possible health).

Analysis

Statistical analysis of the control and treatment groups measured variance (ANOVA, analysis of variance) between the groups at entry, baseline and outcome. It was found that there were more 'urgent referrals' to the treatment group. Further analysis of variance was required to determine whether the difference between the two groups had any effect on outcome. t-tests were used to examine the degree of difference within each group over the course of the study and between the two groups. The study aimed to identify changes in SF–36 scores between 5 (clinically and socially significant) and 10 points (moderate effect).

Results

There was a variable response rate to the outcome questionnaire with a 67% non-response rate in the control group compared to 17.5% non-response in the treatment group. This was dealt with by using a sensitivity analysis to assess the potential for bias (see section on sensitivity analysis, p. 123, in Ch. 10, Systematic reviews). However, the majority of the control group (94%) went on to have treatment, discounting the suggestion that their conditions had improved sufficiently to no longer require treatment.

The analysis had to account for the variability in response between the groups to the questionnaire and the differences identified between the groups (more urgent referrals in treatment group).

ANOVA and *t*-tests established significant differences between the health status of the two groups. Those in the treatment arm scored between 5 and 20 points higher on the SF–36 in seven of the eight scales. The comparison between the groups on the physical functioning scale did not show a significant difference.

manipulated by the researcher as they are already in the past. For example, the researcher may want to explore whether there is a relationship between vaccinations for measles, mumps and rubella (MMR) in childhood and eczema in adults.

Retrospective studies draw on historical data sets which may be problematic when the data have been collected for purposes other than the research, but they can be used when the crucial variable, such as an event like a trauma, has already taken place. Although the aims may be similar to experimental design, retrospective research produces less-convincing evidence of causal relationships between variables.

REGRESSION TO THE MEAN

This refers to the tendency for extreme test scores (pain or other symptoms) to move back towards the group average over time, regardless of whether there has been any intervention or not. The selection process to enter patients into a study may be based on a high scoring of their symptoms. The tendency for the most extreme scores to level out on retesting (with or without treatment) can skew the results. This regression to the mean can be erroneously attributed to the influence of the experimental intervention. In studies comparing one treatment to another this is not a problem, as both groups will be subject to this effect. It is more

Example 8.4   Matched control group (Bagnel et al 1990)

Aim
The aim of this study was to compare the survival and metastasis-free survival of patients treated at the Bristol Cancer Help Centre (BCHC) and a matched control group.

Design
This was a prospectively matched cohort study with outcomes assessed 2 years after recruitment of the first patient. A sample was recruited of 344 women with breast cancer attending the BCHC for the first time. The matched control group was women with breast cancer attending either a specialist NHS cancer centre or one of two participating NHS general hospitals. The control group was stratified into four groups by age and the year of diagnosis and matches taking account of this stratification were selected at random.

Those attending the BCHC were exposed to advice on special diets, counselling and complementary therapies. The matched group received conventional NHS management.

Outcomes were assessed by survival and metastasis-free survival rates 2 years after the first patient was recruited into the study.

Results
Those attending the BCHC had a higher recurrence of metastasis and mortality rate than the control group.

Discussion
Debate following the publication of the paper led to the authors withdrawing their main conclusion that BCHC patients had poorer outcomes than the control group. This was because the matching process was shown to be inadequate and the two groups were shown to be different in important respects. Those attending the BCHC had a higher rate of local recurrence of the disease prior to entering the study. Local recurrence is known to lead to poorer outcomes in breast cancer and this was not controlled for in the matching process. Because the two groups were dissimilar in crucial respects, the original conclusions were invalidated. This underlines the importance of careful matching and also why randomisation at entry has become such a highly valued feature of trial design. Of course it is not always possible or ethical to randomise and so matched groups will continue to be used, but the possibility that the matched groups are systematically different must be borne in mind.

of a problem when the baseline of symptoms is not stable and there is no comparison group.

CAUSATION

Outside the tightly controlled environment of the laboratory, explanatory or fastidious randomised controlled trials provide the most convincing evidence of causal relationships between variables. Using various techniques for reducing bias, such as 'blinding' and controlling for confounding variables through randomisation, the researcher can go further than implying a correlation between variables. The pragmatic trial can show the difference between groups receiving one treatment or another but cannot specify the precise variable that brings about the change. A correlational study may show a link between poverty and heart disease by comparing matched populations but, without the control of the laboratory or a fastidious RCT, establishing cause and effect is very difficult (Bagnel et al 1990).

ADVANTAGES
✔   Useful for getting precise answers to clearly formulated questions
✔   Clear measures for eliminating selection and observation bias
✔   Repeatability. The controlled conditions and pre-specified variables make it possible for other researchers to replicate the study
✔   High credibility in the scientific community

DISADVANTAGES
✗   All the key variables must be understood and included at the design stage. This requires a sound knowledge of the area being investigated
✗   Creating an appropriate outcome measure for the experiment (if a suitable one is not available off the shelf) is likely to require considerable development work
✗   Because all the variables are pre-set, there is little scope for adaptation or exploration once the study is underway
✗   The potential for confounding factors in field experiments is great. The range of safeguards described for RCTs mitigates against confounding factors, but such an undertaking is likely to be beyond the scope of a small-scale researcher
✗   Locating an appropriate population, gaining ethical approval for conducting an experiment, finding willing and available participants from an appropriately chosen sample as well as conducting the experiments and follow-up evaluations takes time. If the researcher is working within time constraints such as those imposed by degree programmes, then it would be unwise to attempt an RCT when so many factors beyond the control of the researcher can lead to delay
✗   A sample that is too small or a degree of change between the groups (intervention and non-intervention) that is small will make it impossible to detect with any degree of statistical confidence the effect of the intervention

References

Bagnel F, Easton D et al 1990 Survival of patients with breast cancer attending Bristol Cancer Help Centre. Lancet **336**: 606–610

Bowling A 1991 Measuring health: a review of quality of life measurement scales. Open University Press, Buckingham

Bowling A 1995 Measuring disease: a review of disease specific quality of life measurement scales. Open University Press, Buckingham

Cardini F, Weixin H 1998 Moxibustion for correction of breech presentation: a randomised controlled trial. Journal of the American Medical Association **280**(18): 1580–1584

Hansen P, Hansen J 1983 Acupuncture treatment of chronic facial pain – a controlled crossover trial. Headache **23**: 66–69

Long A, Mercer G et al 2000 Developing a tool to measure holistic practice: a missing dimension in outcomes measurement within complementary therapies. Complementary Therapies in Medicine **8**: 26–31

Meade T, Dyer S et al 1990 Low back pain of mechanical origin: a randomised comparison of chiropractic and hospital outpatient treatment. British Medical Journal **300**: 349–351

Paterson C 1996 Measuring outcomes in primary care: a patient generated measure, MYMOP, compared with the SF–36 health survey. British Medical Journal **312**: 1016–1020

Reilly D, Taylor M et al 1986 Is homeopathy a placebo response? Controlled trial of homeopathic potency, with pollen in hayfever as model. Lancet **ii**: 881–886

Reuther I, Aldridge D 1998 Qigong Yangsheng as a complementary therapy in the management of asthma: a single-case appraisal. Journal of Alternative and Complementary Medicine **4**(2): 173–183

RIchardson J 1995 Complementary therapies in the NHS: a service evaluation of the first year of an outpatient service in a local district general hospital. The Lewisham Hospital NHS Trust, London

Richardson J 2001a Developing and evaluating complementary therapy services: Part 1. Establishing service provision through the use of evidence and consensus development. Journal of Alternative and Complementary Medicine **7**(3): 253–260

RIchardson J 2001b Developing and evaluating complementary therapy services: Part 2. Examining the effects of treatment on health status. Journal of Alternative and Complementary Medicine **7**(4): 315–328

Vincent C 1990 The treatment of tension headache by acupuncture: a controlled single case design with time series analysis. Journal of Psychosomatic Research **34**(5): 553–561

White A, Ernst E 2001 The case for uncontrolled clinical trials: a starting point for the evidence base for CAM. Complementary Therapies in Medicine **9**(2): 111–116

Surveys

9

INTRODUCTION

The use of surveys is pervasive. One only has to pick up a newspaper to see the results of surveys proclaiming statistics that one in 12 women will have cancer at some time in their lives, that we all live longer and that on average men die 5 years younger than women. Statistics from surveys abound and are much loved by the marketing industry. Just about all of us will have at some time been stopped by an interviewer on a street corner or received through the post a survey asking our opinions on one product or another. The claim that research shows that 'most women prefer Frizzle washing powder' is probably no more than marketing hype and to be taken with a pinch of salt but surveys have a serious use and a long and venerable history. The field of epidemiology, which studies the patterns of health and disease across whole populations, utilises large surveys to make links between disease and our environment, diet or any other factor that may be associated with the disease.

Surveys are used to describe accurately the characteristics of a population, providing information on the distribution of and relationship between those characteristics.

Surveys are an efficient and relatively straightforward way of finding out about people's attitudes, opinions, beliefs, preferences, and behaviours. Whilst not particularly suited to exploratory work or establishing causal relationships, surveys are a useful mapping device. Unlike experimental designs surveys have no interventions or planned changes, and there is none of the detailed background and contextual information that is so important in case studies. Surveys are characterised by the collection of small amounts of data in a standardised format, typically from a large sample.

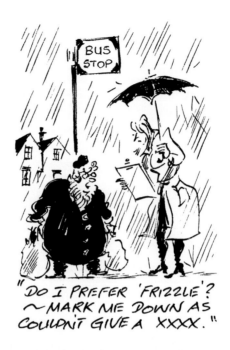

"DO I PREFER 'FRIZZLE'?
~MARK ME DOWN AS
COULDN'T GIVE A XXXX."

> *Surveys are best at telling us* what is there *rather than* how *or* why it
> got there.

METHODS OF SURVEYING

Self-completion questionnaires

POSTAL DISTRIBUTION

Often the most practical way of gathering data from a large set of people over
a short period of time, the postal questionnaire is relatively low-cost and
straightforward to administer. This is a real advantage when the population is
spread out over a wide geographical region and face-to-face interviews would
be time-consuming and costly. The anonymity associated with not having to
meet a researcher face-to-face can help some people to be more frank in
response to questions about sensitive issues. People respond when they choose,
having time to think without the pressure of having to give an immediate
response to questions. There is, however, always the issue that respondents will
not necessarily disclose accurately their beliefs, attitudes or behaviours. This
may be because they do not remember accurately, are unwilling to be seen in
a bad light, do not take the exercise seriously or have misunderstood the
question. Unlike in face-to-face interviews, the researcher has no way of
judging how serious people are being with their responses, or checking out
ambiguities and misunderstandings.

Surveys often rely on what people say they do. Such self-reported behaviour may not be an accurate reflection of what respondents actually do. The response rate to postal surveys can be very low. The fact that they are mostly sent 'cold', without any personal contact, is probably a factor in this low response rate. Other factors, such as the relevance of the topic to respondents, the number of questions and the ease with which they can be understood, will all influence response rate.

Once the initial work on developing the questionnaire and locating a sample is complete, a postal survey can provide a large volume of data fairly rapidly for analysis.

Because the format for response is standardised, analysis is relatively simple and typically amenable to statistical analysis. Cassidy's (1998a,b) survey of Chinese medicine use in a US population is described in Example 9.1. For a more detailed discussion on questionnaire design and implementation, see Chapter 13, Questionnaires.

DIRECT DISTRIBUTION

This may be via a central point of contact for the population in question, such as a clinic, service centre, shop or other outlet. If a representative sample is being sought it is crucial that all members of the identified population are given an equal opportunity to participate — see Chapter 11, Sampling, for further discussion on this issue.

EMAIL SURVEY

Sharing many of the characteristics of postal questionnaires, email surveys can be sent out to a population with a wide geographical spread for next to no cost. It may be difficult, however, to calculate exactly who or how many will be contacted through a mailshot. It is also important that relevant members of the population are not excluded because they are not online. Some groups, such as the elderly or unemployed, may be excluded because of a lack of access to the internet. The fact that there are no envelopes to be posted makes replying simpler and in principle should encourage a higher response rate.

Interviews

The smiling market researcher with clipboard in hand is a familiar sight in shopping centres. One of the reasons interviews are so popular is that the personal contact encourages the participation of respondents. This personal approach is helpful in other ways. As well as explaining to respondents why they should participate in the research, the researcher can also clarify the survey questions if the responses suggest that the question has not been understood. This ability to respond on the ground is an advantage over postal questionnaires. The response rate tends to be better than with postal surveys as the researcher can sell the point of the research. When there is a requirement for certain quotas, for instance age, gender, etc., the researcher's attention can be directed to meeting these quotas.

Example 9.1 Survey (Cassidy 1998a, 1998b)

This survey of Chinese medicine usage in a US population has been divided and published in two parts. The first part reports the quantitative findings and the second the qualitative findings.

Aim
To document the usage of Chinese medicine in a US population and record users' opinions and experiences of the care they received.

Design
Qualitative and quantitative in-depth survey based on a written questionnaire.

Sampling
Participating clinics were selected purposively, based on offering comprehensive care, urban and suburban location and large patient flow (greater that 80 per week). Of eight centres identified as meeting these criteria, six agreed to participate. Over a scheduled 14-day collection period just under 45.9% of those patients invited agreed to participate, leading to a total of 575 completed questionnaires.

Data collection
Quantitative data were collected on user demographics, reasons for choosing Chinese medicine, particular modalities of treatment used (i.e. acupuncture, herbs, diet, etc.), response to treatment and user satisfaction.

Qualitative data were collected based on written responses to survey questions.

Analysis
Descriptive statistics were developed for the quantitative section using the software Statistical Package for the Social Sciences (SPSS).

Qualitative data were collated using the software Ethnograph and analysed in terms of themes running through the data set and in relation to an overarching concept of holism. The conceptual framework was based on concepts of holism as articulated through the literature in this field.

Results

Quantitative data provided a demographic picture of the users as mid-aged, well-educated, employed, mid-income patients seeking care for a wide variety of conditions including musculoskeletal pain, emotional support and support for wellbeing. A majority reported improvement of symptoms and expressed a high level of satisfaction with the Chinese medical care they received.

Qualitative data presented excerpts of patient stories as well as general themes about relief of symptoms, improved function and coping ability. These themes were embedded in an analysis of how the Chinese medical care these users received was addressing contemporary 'home grown' concerns for genuinely holistic health care, as opposed to the seeking of Chinese medicine because it was exotic or foreign.

Although the personal contact encourages participation and potentially leads to richer data than a postal questionnaire, there are downsides. One of the most important is the cost in terms of the researcher's time spent interviewing and travelling to interview sites. There is also the question about whether the personal characteristics of the researcher (age, race, gender, personality) may unwittingly bias how people respond. The reduced sense of anonymity compared to a postal questionnaire may lead to less honest or open responses. There is also the question about how careful and accurate the responses are likely to be in a fleeting interaction with a stranger.

TELEPHONE INTERVIEWS

Telephone interviews have become an increasingly popular research tool as they are cheaper and quicker to conduct than face-to-face interviews, with some of the same advantages (Eisenburg et al 1993). With a personal touch the researcher can explain why the research is being conducted and encourage respondents to participate. Questions can be clarified when it is doubtful that the respondent has fully understood what was meant. There are compromises, however; the interviewer cannot pick up on important non-verbal data as in face-to-face interviews, but this disadvantage needs to be offset by the considerable savings made in time and travel. Although making contact is easy by telephone, there is a higher refusal rate than with postal questionnaires, perhaps because telephone calls can be quite intrusive and inconvenient. In an era when more than 90% of the adult population are contactable by phone, former concerns about ensuring a representative sample are diminishing and the argument that people are less likely to be honest than in face-to-face interviews has not been supported by research investigating this question. When working with large populations, computer technology can be used to dial random numbers within a designated dialling code area, aiding in the sampling process.

Documents

Although questionnaires and interviews are the most common methods used in survey research, there are projects that can utilise documents and observations rather than direct questioning of individuals. If the research question is concerned with medical notes or written policy guidelines, then a key source of data would be an examination of the documents themselves.

Observations

The geographical survey uses direct observation to get the 'lay of the land'. In health-related research it is possible to survey the physical characteristics of an environment; for instance, if one is interested in the ergonomic characteristics of a workplace, direct observation at a series of sites would be the main data source. Behaviours might also be the focus of observation: to stay with the ergonomic example, it might be lifting practices utilised by nurses. What would make these kinds of observations useful for survey research is how the data are collected. A standardised format for the collection of small amounts of data utilising a large sample will allow meaningful comparisons to be made within the data set, and generalisations to be made about the entire population (see Ch. 14, Observations).

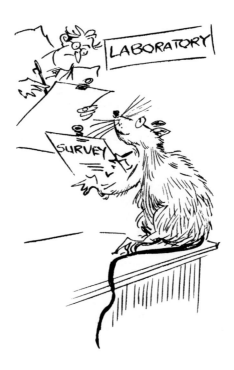

Small amounts of data utilising a large sample characterise surveys.

RESPONSE RATES

The level of response will depend on many factors, such as the nature of the respondents and the subject of the research. Surveys of 20–35-year-olds typically have a lower response rate than surveys of the over-65s, who are likely to be retired and have more time to respond to surveys. But more important than the question of time is whether the research topic seems relevant. A survey of preferred contraception methods may not grab the attention of the over-80s, just as satisfaction with a home health care service may not interest an under-20s population. How the survey is presented will also affect response rate, i.e. whether in written form or by an interviewer. A range of social determinants might be important, such as gender, race, age, etc. With postal questionnaires reminders can be sent to all non-responders.

There are no hard and fast rules about what constitutes a good response rate. One can check the response rate with other comparable surveys. In most fields a response rate of 70% and above is considered good and greater than 60% quite acceptable.

REPRESENTATIVENESS

Whether through non-contact or refusal, a non-response rate of, say, greater than 25% calls into question whether those who did not respond had shared characteristics. From any representative sample it is likely that some people cannot be contacted and some may be unwilling to participate. There is also a good chance that the excluded members will not be representative of the sample. This needs to be checked out whenever possible, as the data set may be biased by this difference. How much of a problem this is depends upon how atypical (in ways that are relevant to the survey) those excluded are. A large non-response rate might not be such a problem if the researcher is only interested in broad trends. On the other hand, if the researcher wanted to know the opinions of different user groups of a service, then a small non-response rate from a minority group would invalidate the findings. This problem may be best dealt with at the design stage by stratifying the sample (see Ch. 11, Sampling). If the problem is only detected after the main survey has been conducted, it may be possible to use a *booster sample*, where an additional sample is taken and the results are added to the main survey. The problem with this is that the booster sample will probably require a different sampling strategy from the main sample (which led to under-representation). What this means is that in effect two different surveys are being added together, leading to problems with statistical analysis.

ADVANTAGES

✔ They provide a straightforward approach to studying opinions, attitudes and behaviours as well as events. The focus may be contemporaneous or relate to the past

✔ The breadth is wide and inclusive, typically based on small amounts of data from a large representative sample. Thus the findings of good survey research can be generalised to the wider population

✔ The responses are typically quantifiable and amenable to statistical analysis – fundamental when making generalisations

✔ The method is structured and systematic in the way data are collected and analysed and this process can be made transparent to those evaluating the research

✔ They are highly adaptable and may be used in a wide range of settings with most populations

✔ A key feature of survey work is its empirical nature, getting out into the field to find out what is there. The focus is upon presenting the data rather than the development of theory or proving causal relationships

✔ The costs associated with surveys are considerably less than most other forms of research

DISADVANTAGES

✘ The quality of the data is dependent upon respondents' characteristics, including the reliability of their memories as well as levels of motivation

✘ A lack of depth and detail occurs when the data analysis is based on average responses to specific questions. Although useful and important for making generalisations, the findings can seem decontextualised

✘ Respondents may not report their personal beliefs or behaviours accurately. This can be dependent upon what they perceive to be the most socially desirable response

✘ Interview data may be unduly influenced by the personality or social characteristics of the interviewer, or by non-verbal cues implying 'correct' answers. An Asian and a neo-fascist skinhead conducting interviews about immigration into the UK are likely to elicit quite different responses

✘ How the questions are framed, and the range of possible responses, are predetermined by the researcher, leaving little scope for respondents to explain or make explicit their own frames of reference

✘ Postal surveys may have low response rates as well as ambiguities and misunderstanding of the survey questions

References

Cassidy C 1998a Chinese medicine users in the United States Part I: utilisation, satisfaction, medical plurality. Journal of Alternative and Complementary Medicine 4(1): 17–27

Cassidy C 1998b Chinese medicine users in the United States Part II: preferred aspects of care. Journal of Alternative and Complementary Medicine 4(2): 189–202

Eisenburg D, Kessler C et al 1993 Unconventional medicine in the United States: prevalence, costs, and patterns of use. New England Journal of Medicine 328(4): 246–252

Systematic reviews

10

WHAT IS A SYSTEMATIC REVIEW?

A systematic review is based upon an explicit and replicable procedure to critically appraise and synthesise the results of all relevant studies that address a specific clinical question. Like all human activities, the literature review is subject to bias. The traditional or what is sometimes called a narrative review paper does not usually state how the authors searched for and identified the studies they cite. The reader is without a basis to judge whether or not the cited studies have been chosen selectively to support the author's own prejudices. It is not too unusual to find a series of positive or negative papers, depending on the author's own prejudices.

Traditional narrative reviews are useful for obtaining a broad perspective on a topic and describing cutting edge work where there is a limited volume of research. They are also appropriate for describing the history or development of a problem and its management. However, the connection between clinical recommendations and evidence in narrative reviews can be incomplete, or — worse still — based on a biased citation of studies.

A systematic review differs from the traditional narrative review by using a transparent and replicable strategy to study the best evidence for an intervention. The use of explicit, systematic methods helps prevent both systematic errors (bias) and random errors (simple mistakes) from creeping into the work. Systematic reviews are generated to answer specific, often narrow, clinical questions, thus providing more reliable results from which to draw conclusions and make decisions (Vernon et al 1999). They can also be used to

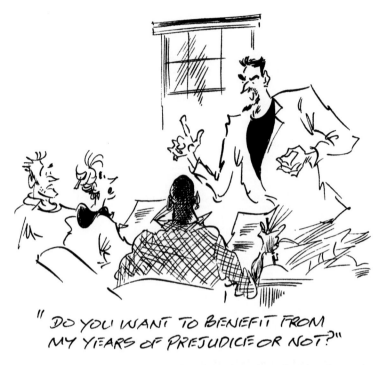

" DO YOU WANT TO BENEFIT FROM
MY YEARS OF PREJUDICE OR NOT?"

answer non-clinical questions such as how prevalent the use of complementary therapies is in a specific population (Ernst & Cassileth 1998, Harris & Rees 2000). Rather than reflecting the views of an 'expert', a systematic review collates and analyses all the relevant studies. Conclusions or recommendations are based on the whole body of relevant evidence. When the results of primary studies are summarised but not statistically combined, the review may be called a narrative systematic review (Vernon et al 1999). It is known as a meta-analysis when statistical methods are used to pool the results of the studies included (Linde et al 1996). Single studies rarely provide definitive answers to clinical questions. Individual research studies may come up with different conclusions, leading to uncertainty for practitioners about the value of an intervention. This is one of the reasons why variations in practice exist. The systematic review can help practitioners make a judgement based on all the relevant studies. It can also highlight the lack of available evidence and can be used as a basis for planning specific research to fill the knowledge gaps.

This chapter draws on the extensive work of the Cochrane Collaboration, an international multidisciplinary collaboration that is working towards systematically reviewing the range of healthcare interventions (http://www.update-software.com/cochrane/).

HOW TO DO IT

The key steps in carrying out a systematic review are given in Box 10.1 and discussed below.

Box 10.1 Key steps in carrying out a systematic review

- Define the focus and breadth of the review (the condition or treatment you are interested in)
- Formulate the precise question the review will ask
- Define the characteristics of the population within primary studies
- Define the intervention
- Define the relevant outcomes
- Define your search strategy for locating relevant studies (published and unpublished)
- Set the inclusion and exclusion criteria for the primary studies
- Data extraction
- Data synthesis (non-statistical and statistical)
- Data analysis
- Data presentation
- Drawing conclusions

Defining the question

Like all scientific investigations a systematic review requires a clearly formulated question to focus the study. You should be able to make a clear statement about what it is you want to find out from the review process. You need to define as precisely as you can the main question that the review is intended to answer. A clearly defined question will make explicit the specific population and setting (such as pre-term infants in a neonatal ward), the condition of interest (such as respiratory distress), the nature of the exposure or intervention (such as aromatherapy) and the kind of outcomes to be considered (such as levels of respiratory distress and antibiotic use). You will also need to make explicit the types of studies relevant to answering your question. They could be randomised controlled trials, case control studies or cohort studies, depending upon the question you have defined. Most of the existing systematic reviews rely heavily on randomised controlled trials (because they address interventions) and some exclude all other kinds of research. The methodology for including qualitative studies in a systematic review is at the present time poorly developed.

If the review is concerned exclusively with effectiveness of interventions as defined by specific outcome measures, it may be that the only studies conforming to this are RCTs. Within some clinical disciplines randomised controlled trials are extremely difficult to set up or altogether inappropriate, and other methods such as case control studies or cohort studies may provide the best currently available evidence. You should take care that your review does not exclude the best current evidence by having inclusion criteria that are excessively narrow. Equally, it is of no value to widen the inclusion criteria to allow low-quality or inappropriate studies to be included. To define the review question, it helps if you have some familiarity with the literature in the field.

See Chapter 8, Experiments and quasi-experiments, for further discussion about randomised controlled trials and their application.

Deciding how broad your research question should be

It may be that you are interested in reviewing an area where there have not been many studies that could be included. In this case you will need to ensure that the research question guiding the review is sufficiently broad. For example, take the question: 'Does St John's wort have a beneficial effect in post-natal depression?' If there are very few studies in this area you may need to broaden the review question to include all studies evaluating St John's wort in depression, as did Linde et al (1996) in their systematic review of St John's wort. To group these conditions together you will want to ensure that there are no grounds for believing that there would be a markedly different response to the intervention in the included conditions.

Having established your research question, you will also need to be clear whether the participants of the primary studies to be included in the review are sufficiently similar. If a treatment is known to have very different effects in the very young and the elderly, then including such studies in the same review will be like trying to evaluate grapes along with raisins.

If you are interested in a condition where the outcomes of treatment are known to vary with age or environment, you will need to account for this and decide how broad your inclusion criteria should be. On the other hand, you should not restrict the population of interest without clear justification.

Box 10.2 lists the questions you should ask when defining your review question.

Box 10.2   Defining the review question

- Is the focus of the question broad or narrow?
- What is the condition you are interested in?
- What is the intervention, therapy or exposure?
- What kinds of participants will have received the intervention?
- What outcomes will you be considering?
- If you are reviewing effectiveness, what are the parameters?
- What kinds of studies will be included in your review?

Locating relevant studies

The aim of the search is to generate as comprehensive a list as possible of primary studies, both published and unpublished, which may be suitable for answering the questions posed in the review.

CHECKING REFERENCE LISTS

Checking the references of key papers is an efficient way of locating relevant research but it is very unlikely to be either complete or comprehensive. Obtain copies of previous reviews, as they will provide a good source of primary studies.

DEFINING THE SEARCH STRATEGY FOR LOCATING RELEVANT STUDIES

Searching the literature has become much easier with powerful electronic databases such as PubMed (MEDLINE), but this will only provide a starting point. Depending upon your field of interest, PubMed may not have all the relevant studies that should be included. Many high-quality studies published in languages other than English will not find their way onto PubMed. This makes it imperative to have a broad search strategy.

When searching databases such as PubMed, include multiple key words to ensure that you do not miss studies. If you are interested in the treatment of neck pain by osteopathy, as well as using the key word neck pain you should also include cervical spine pain. As well as using osteopathy you should include manipulation, physiotherapy, chiropractic and manual medicine. By using the word 'or' between the above words you will locate any papers containing these key words. (See Ch. 3, Reviewing the literature, for a simplified example of a database search strategy.) Harris and Rees' (2000) review of the prevalence of complementary therapy use made searches of the MEDLINE and CISCOM databases (see Example 10.1).

Example 10.1   Systematic review (Harris & Rees 2000)

Aim

This review examined the prevalence of complementary and alternative medicine use in the general populations of Australia, Canada, Finland, Israel, the UK and USA.

Method

Searches were undertaken using the terms 'alternative medicine' and 'health care surveys' in two bibliographic databases — MEDLINE and CISCOM (a specialised database for complementary medicine) — for all years up to 1999. Further attempts to locate papers were made by examining citations in the papers found within the initial search.

Papers were included in the review if they met all three of the following criteria:

- survey methods (structured interviews or self-completed questionnaires) were used to estimate the extent of complementary medicine usage among a target population
- usage was measured among the general population rather than in specific sub-groups

---

continued overpage

continued

- the prevalence was measured as a percentage of the general population.

Papers were excluded if any of the following criteria were met:
- estimates of prevalence were single therapy only (e.g. homeopathy)
- study methods were insufficiently described
- the report was not written in English.

Substantive information, such as date of survey administration, target population, therapies listed and estimated prevalence, was recorded along with how papers fared in relation to inclusion and exclusion criteria.

Methodological issues

A total of 638 references were found, of these only 12 met the study inclusion criteria. The methodological quality of the remaining 12 papers was evaluated and it was found that important methodological information was missing in some of the papers, such as sampling method (two papers failed to report this and three stated that random samples were used, but the randomisation process was not described). Three of the studies failed to specify their response rate. None of the studies provided a clear rationale for the number and type of therapies included in their definitions of complementary and alternative medicine. Only two of the studies checked the reliability of the responses provided in the surveys by following up 5% of the sample with interviews. Although nine of the 12 studies described their findings as representative or generalisable to the target population, only six supported the claim with some evidence.

Findings

The most rigorous studies conducted in Australia and USA found that near to half of the population had used non-medically prescribed alternative medicine and 12–20% had visited practitioners of complementary/alternative medicine.

CITATION INDEXES

A citation search can be a useful way of locating studies. This is where you identify a key paper and then search for other papers that have included this key paper in their references. Online databases such as SCISEARCH and BIDS perform this specific function very simply. (See Ch. 3, Reviewing the literature, for more detail on citation indexes.)

THE COCHRANE LIBRARY

This has three databases of published and ongoing systematic reviews:
- **The Cochrane Database of Systematic Reviews (CDSR)** contains the full text of regularly updated systematic reviews of the effects of health care carried out by the Cochrane collaboration, plus

protocols for reviews currently in preparation (available at http://www.update-software.com/cochrane/).

- **The Database of Abstracts of Reviews of Effectiveness (DARE)** contains critical appraisals of systematic reviews not published in the CDSR. These reviews are identified by regular searching of bibliographic databases, hand searching of key major medical journals, and by scanning 'grey literature' (conference proceedings, dissertations etc.) (DARE is also available at http://www.york.ac.uk/inst/crd).

- **The Health Technology Assessment (HTA) Database** contains abstracts of completed technology assessments and ongoing projects being conducted by members of the International Network of Agencies for Health Technology Assessment (INAHTA) and other healthcare technology agencies (HTA database is also available at http://www.york.ac.uk/inst/crd).

The following software is available for performing systematic reviews and meta-analysis:

- Mulrow C, Oxman A (eds) (1997) **The Cochrane Collaboration Handbook** (CD-ROM), The Cochrane Library. Oxford Update Software — for members of the collaboration

- **Meta-Stat 1.5** — free software from www.download.com (for PCs only)

- **Comprehensive Meta-Analysis** commercial software from www.meta-analysis.com

There are also various registers of research, such as the National Register of Research in the UK (http://www.update-software.com/). On this site trials are registered at inception rather than following publication, providing valuable information on work in progress, or possibly on publication bias when completed studies are not published.

PERSONAL COMMUNICATION

Colleagues, researchers and educators in the field may be able to tell you about current trials that have not yet been published or older trials that were never published. There may be a significant grey literature in the form of conference proceedings, dissertations and technical reports that you may be able to locate. If this literature does not contain sufficient detail to include in your data analysis, you could contact the authors who may be willing to provide the detail you require.

HAND SEARCHING

There may be specialist libraries in your field that you could visit and hand search for relevant publications. As with all forms of searching you are likely to experience diminishing returns for your search efforts, and just how much time you can spend doing this will depend upon deadlines and available resources. Specialist librarians may be able to help point you towards the relevant publications.

Defining and refining inclusion and exclusion criteria for studies

It is sensible to test the inclusion criteria on a sample of articles (say 6–10 papers, including ones that are thought to be definitely eligible, definitely not eligible and questionable). The pilot test can be used to refine and clarify the inclusion criteria. These criteria should be explicit so that they may be applied consistently by more than one person. In areas where you have some expertise you are likely to have some pre-formed opinions that may bias your judgement about the relevance and validity of articles. It may be advantageous to have a second reviewer, who is not an expert in the area, review a sample of articles to establish congruence.

Audit trail

It is important to report in sufficient detail how the search was conducted so that another investigator could replicate your search. This is part of the transparency that allows the reader to judge whether or not your review has included or omitted studies that might bias your findings. Your trail should include the main sources that were used to locate the studies, the specific search strategies used for each database you searched, including key words and the dates searched. A much simplified example follows in Box 10.3.

Box 10.3   Audit trail

PubMed (MEDLINE), EMBASE and CISCOM databases were searched for articles published between 1970 and 2001. Key words used were:
(Neck pain or cervical spine pain and osteopathy or manipulation or physiotherapy or chiropractic or manual medicine) and (randomised controlled trial or clinical trial or placebo controlled trial).

Managing and coding the data

All the papers selected should be kept on a reference management system such as EndNote (for Mac OS 9, Mac OS X and PC), Reference Manager (PC only) or ProCite (PC and Mac OS 9). These software applications will help you to manage and organise your growing data set. Reference sets from online databases such as PubMed can be downloaded directly into software application. They can be used to check whether there is duplication in the data set when different search methods come up with the same references. Another important check is to ensure that data from the same patients are not included more than once. A data set should only be included once, whether it has been presented in various publications or not.

DESIGNING A STUDY INCLUSION FORM

Once you obtain either the abstracts or complete copies of the papers identified through the search, you will need to make a judgement about each paper to decide whether it should be included in the review. The abstract is mostly adequate to judge whether the paper meets the inclusion criteria; however, if you are unsure from the abstract, then the full paper must be examined. A study inclusion or in/out form is a basic checklist to establish whether a paper should be included in the review. This should be kept quite simple, with basic data on the population, intervention and methodology. An example from Little and Parsons' (2001) review on the use of herbal preparations for arthritis is given in Figure 10.1.

DATA EXTRACTION (Study Inclusion)

(please circle)   INCLUDE, level 1 EXCLUDE   PENDING

IDENTIFICATION: Reference:_____   Paper ID: _____   Study ID ____   Reviewer: _____

CRITERIA (please circle response)	Met	Not Met
1. Human, not animal, study	YES	NO → exclude
2. Is there a formal diagnosis of arthritis[1]?	YES	NO → exclude
3. Was a herbal preparation[2] administered to the intervention group?	YES	NO → exclude
Did the preparation include any non-herbal substance[3]?	NO	YES → exclude
4. Did the control group receive a placebo?	YES	No → exclude
5. Did author(s) state that subjects were randomised[4] to either		
intervention or control groups?	YES	NO → exclude

● if 'yes' to criteria 1–5 → include   if 'unsure' to any criterion → pending

If paper fails to meet all inclusion criteria, please elaborate upon reasons (continue overleaf):

---

[1]Diagnosis. All types of arthritis to be included (rheumatoid arthritis, osteoarthritis, psoriatic arthritis, juvenile arthritis etc.). Broad descriptions of the population (e.g. 'joint pain', 'amavata'), without a formal diagnosis of arthritis, should be excluded

[2]Herbal preparation. Herbal medicine, or phytotherapy, relates to the use of natural source, whole plant extracts. Include studies that describe any type of Western, Oriental, or other, herbal preparation. Exclude studies that describe homeopathy, aromatherapy, plant derivative (i.e. not whole plant), synthetic derivative

[3]Non-herbal substance. Studies should be excluded where the intervention includes any substance of non-herbal origin except where the purpose of the non-herbal substance is clearly stated to be for reasons other than treatment of the condition. (E.g. the addition of vitamin E as an anti-oxidant would be acceptable)

[4]Randomisation. Any mention of random, randomly or randomisation in reference to allocation of groups is acceptable

Figure 10.1   Study inclusion form (from Little & Parsons 2001 with permission of the authors).

DESIGNING A DATA EXTRACTION FORM

You should design an electronic or paper form that will allow you to code each section of the included papers, with space for comments and judgements.

The categories and criteria will depend to some extent upon the research question, but if the review is an evaluation of a healthcare intervention then you will need to include sections on methods, participants, interventions and outcomes. The criteria within each section should be explicit. A great deal of work has been done on critically evaluating research, and you will need to be familiar with the issues related to the field of study you interested in. Many of the important issues have been discussed in other chapters of this book. You can also find out more by checking out the Cochrane Library at http://www.update-software.com/cochrane/.

SELECTION OF STUDIES AND DATA EXTRACTION

When you have coded all the studies you will have to make a judgement as to which ones to include in the review. This will depend upon the question the review is attempting to answer and the methodological quality of the studies found. The criteria used for judging the methodological quality of individual studies will depend upon whether they are randomised controlled trials, case control studies, observational studies, etc. Chapter 8, Experiments and quasi-experiments, will help you to understand these.

You should carefully extract the data from the primary studies in their original form before reworking them so that all the studies can be considered together.

The following example of a data extraction form (Fig. 10.2) is from the systematic review on herbal interventions in arthritis by Little and Parsons (2001). The precise features that are relevant will depend upon the question the review is attempting to answer, but an evaluation of a healthcare intervention is likely to have a similar list of questions.

Methods

The methods section of the data extraction form should include: data on type of study, e.g. parallel or cross-over design; methods of randomisation and allocation concealment, e.g. patient, provider and outcome assessor blinding; number of drop-outs and cross-overs; co-interventions and other potential confounding factors that will depend upon the study design.

Participants

As participants may vary from study to study, it is important to identify characteristics that could lead to significant differences in outcome. This might include age and gender for certain clinical conditions. Concurrent illnesses can affect clinical outcomes, as may length of time the participant has had the condition being studied. If the environment in which the condition occurs or the treatment given is likely to be a significant factor, this should be identified. For example, an intervention of healthcare advice given in a hospital and in the community may be received and acted on in very different ways, resulting in quite different outcomes.

Interventions

Details about the intervention should be recorded, including the mode of administration, the dosage and the length of time given. If a placebo control group was used, information on how the placebo was administered should also be recorded.

DATA EXTRACTION
PLEASE CIRCLE RESPONSES AND ADD COMMENTS WHERE NECESSARY

10. KEY: T = Treatment group   C = Control group
                SUMMARY (please complete once data extraction has been completed)

11. Y = Yes   N = No   Un = Uncertain
    Results favour: Intervention   Control   Equivocal
    N/A = Not applicable   * = please specify

                              FUNDING
IDENTIFICATION
12.   Source of funding identified?   Yes* _____

                                             No _____
Author(s) _____
Reference _____

                             MISSING DATA
Data missing from any section?   Yes[1]   →   Section(s) _____
                                      No
[1]Is any of this information required? Yes[2]   →   Section(s) _____
                                      No
Paper ID _____ Study ID _____
Study location _____   Year of study _____
[2]Has author been contacted?   Yes[3]
                                                     No
[3]How was author contacted?   e-mail   letter   telephone
[3]How did author respond?   e-mail   letter   telephone no response

Source MEDLINE EMBASE CISCOM AMED CINAHL CTTR BIDS ISI SIGLE DISS AB Un

              Comments (please refer to section[s] as appropriate)

Figure 10.2   Data extraction form (from Little & Parsons 2001 with permission of the authors).

Outcomes

You need to be clear about what kind of outcome data will help you answer the question guiding the review. Different studies looking at the same intervention may use different outcome measures recorded at different times. You will need to integrate this information in light of the review question.

Table 10.1 Methodological quality of surveys of complementary and alternative medicine use (from Harris and Rees 2000 with permission of Elsevier)

Author place	Survey mode	n	Sampling methods	Response rate (%)	Sample size calculation?	Rationale for therapy choice and question wording	Reliability of survey assessed	Data examined/ adjusted for representativeness?
MacLennan et al 1996 Australia	Face-to-face interview	3004	Systematic sampling of districts, random selection of households, selection of respondents not specified	73	Sample size calculated	NS	NS	Data weighted by age, gender and geographical region to the 1991 South Australian Census
Verhoef et al 1994 Canada	Face-to-face interview	563	NS	78	NS	NS	NS	Sample considered to be similar to rural population of Alberta (no detail)

Millar 1997 Canada	Face-to-face interview	17626	NS (cites reports)	NS	NS	NS	NS	Data age adjusted based on estimated 1994 Canadian population (no detail)
Vaskilampi et al 1993 Finland	Telephone interview	1618	Stratified random sample from Census Bureau	92	NS	Refers to pilot studies (no detail)	NS	Compares sample with government statistics on a range of sociodemographic variables
Bernstein & Shuval 1997 Israel	Face-to-face interview	2030	Random sample (no detail)	NS	NS	NS	NS	Representative sample (no detail)
Yung et al 1988 UK	Self-complete questionnaire	4268	Systematic random sample from electoral register	70	NS	NS	NS	Respondents do not differ from 1981 census data for same area (no detail)

continued over page

continued

Author place	Survey mode	n	Sampling methods	Response rate (%)	Sample size calculation?	Rationale for therapy choice and question wording	Reliability of survey assessed	Data examined/ adjusted for representa- tiveness?
Thomas et al 1993 UK	Self-complete questionnaire	676	Systematic random sample from electoral register	73	NS	Describes pilot study	5% of sample checked	Compares age and gender to 1991 OPCS General Household Survey
Eisenberg et al 1993 USA	Telephone interview	1539	Random digit dialling to select households, random selection of respondent within household	67	Sample size calculated	Refers to pilot studies (no detail)	5% of sample checked (no results given)	Compares sample with 1989 National Health Interview Survey on a range of sociodemo- graphic variables
Eisenberg et al 1998 USA	Telephone interview	2055	Ditto above with further random sample of initial refusals	60	Sample size calculated	Replicates 1993 study	NS	Compares sample with US Census on a range of sociodemographic variables

Paramore 1997 USA	Telephone interview	3450	National probability sample (no detail)	75	NS	NS	NS	Estimates weighted to US civilian, non-institutionalised population (no detail)
Burg et al 1998 USA	Telephone interview	1012	Random digit dialling to select households, stratified by region	54	NS	Investigator judgement	NS	Sample representative of Florida population for sex, race and annual household income
Landmark Healthcare 1998 USA	Telephone interview	1500	Random sample of households (no detail)	NS	NS	NS	NS	Compares age, ethnicity and education of sample to 1990 US Census

NS = not specified.

Data analysis

DESCRIPTIVE OR NARRATIVE ANALYSIS OF SYSTEMATIC REVIEW

A descriptive analysis details the different studies and summarises the key points. The most accessible way of presenting this is in a table. The table should provide a summary of the evidence of each study and a judgement on the methodological rigour. You will have to decide what comparisons to make and then summarise the comparisons in a table. Table 10.1 is from the study by Harris and Rees (2000).

The next step is to systematically investigate the differences and make a judgement about the effect of the intervention across the studies. The crucial questions that must be addressed are listed in Box 10.4.

Box 10.4   Questions for consideration

1.   What comparisons should be made?
2.   What results should be used in each comparison?
3.   How similar are the results within each comparison?
4.   How can you best summarise the effects for each comparison?
5.   How reliable are those summaries?

STATISTICS OR NOT?

The purpose of a systematic review is to evaluate and summarise the results of all the studies in the area. An important step in this is to see how consistent the results are among the included studies; if they are not, you will need to analyse why this is the case. This process of collating and summarising the findings may be done with statistics or without, but there are cautions whichever approach is used. The basis of the summary and analysis depends upon having information on:

- key variables that characterise the participants
- key variables that characterise the interventions
- key variables that characterise the outcome measures
- results — preferably in a standardised format.

META-ANALYSIS

Meta-analysis is the use of statistics to integrate the results of the included studies. A meta-analysis is a powerful way of evaluating the effects of an intervention. However, the desire to come up with a final conclusion expressed as a few numbers may obscure the complexity of the real world situation. The populations, interventions and outcome measures of the studies included in the review may differ in important ways that prevent meaningful statistical aggregation. In such cases analysis may be better expressed in a non-statistical narrative summary. On the other hand, the simple counting of positive or negative studies by itself is inadequate, small but important changes may be overlooked in a single study. A small change and small sample size may lead to insufficient statistical power to determine whether the changes were due to random factors. The study may report that there were no significant results and be described as a negative study. Combining the data in a meta-analysis may clarify whether those changes were due to the intervention or to random factors. The other problem with simple vote counting of positive and negative studies is when equal weight is given to all the included studies without regard for the size and quality of each study. Larger studies are often more reliable, being less prone to random error and publication bias. Weighting different studies based on the strength of their evidence requires judgement and should be based on explicit criteria.

You should not attempt a meta-analysis if the relevant valid data are lacking. You may not find this out until all the data have been collected. Data from poor or marginal quality studies must be excluded. If the studies are too dissimilar or the populations are heterogeneous, meta-analysis may be inappropriate. In these cases a narrative analysis can explore how the differences in study characteristics affect the results. As a rule, if it is not clear how a meta-analysis will help answer the questions guiding the review, you are better not using this technique.

TABULATING STATISTICAL DATA

There is a range of statistical tests that can be applied to the data to explore the differences between participants, interventions and outcome measures.

If you have no background in statistics, guidance from a statistician will be invaluable. There are several software packages specifically designed for performing meta-analysis and some of these are detailed on page 113, earlier in the chapter. While it is not necessary to be competent in the mathematics of statistical analysis, an understanding of basic concepts and how to input the data is needed. Different kinds of data require different statistical treatment. Chapter 17, Analysing quantitative data, provides an introduction to the basics, but you should take expert advice on the choice of statistical tests.

SENSITIVITY ANALYSIS

There is a range of methods you may use to test the robustness of the results of your systematic review. Sensitivity analysis involves repeating the analysis whilst making small changes to the data. By examining the key decisions you make in selecting and analysing the primary data, you should be able to convince yourself (and the reader of your review) that your results are an accurate representation of the data rather than an artefact of your method.

You should consider whether changing the inclusion criteria would have a substantive effect on your results; consider types of participants, interventions and outcome measures, excluding unpublished studies or studies of lower methodological quality and reanalysing the data using different statistical techniques.

If the results of your data synthesis are not significantly altered when any of the above criteria are extended, then you can have greater confidence in your interpretations and conclusions. If, on the other hand, the results are altered by extending the inclusion criteria, you will need to exercise caution in drawing conclusions and to attempt some analysis of why these differences exist.

Presenting your report

An example of the structure of a systematic review report is given in Box 10.5.

Box 10.5   Suggested structure of a systematic review report

Title
Summary or structured abstract
Context
Objectives
Methods (data sources, study selection, quality assessment and data extraction)
Results (data synthesis)
Conclusions
Main text
Background
Questions addressed by the review (hypotheses tested)
Review methods (how the research was conducted)
Data sources and search strategy
Study selection (inclusion and exclusion criteria)
Study quality assessment
Data extraction
Data synthesis
Details of the included and excluded studies
Results of the review
Findings of the review
Robustness of the results (sensitivity analysis)
Discussion (interpretation of results)
Conclusions
Recommendations for health care
Implications for further research
Acknowledgements
Conflict of interest
References
Appendices
(Based on guidelines created by NHS Centre for Research and Dissemination, University of York, www.york.ac.uk/inst/crd)

ADVANTAGES

✔ Uses an explicit and replicable procedure to critically appraise and synthesise the results of all relevant studies that address a specific clinical question

✔ Systematic and clearly articulated methods help prevent both systematic errors (bias) and random errors (simple mistakes) from creeping into the work

✔ Conclusions or recommendations are based on the whole body of relevant evidence. A traditional or narrative review is subject to the unspecified bias of the author

DISADVANTAGES

✘ Systematic reviews are designed to answer specific, often narrow, questions, typically on the efficacy of an intervention

✘ Systematic reviews rely on there being a sufficient body of high-quality studies to draw on. Methodological difficulties or economic constraints mean only a small number of high-quality studies (particularly RCTs) have been conducted in the field of complementary medicine

✘ If the selection criteria for studies are too narrow, the best available evidence may be excluded from the review (for instance patient and evaluator blinding to the intervention, which is problematic when hands-on techniques like bodywork are used)

✘ Conducting a thorough systematic review is not a soft option for research. It takes a lot of time to design, conduct and analyse

References

Bernstein JH, Shuval JT 1997 Nonconventional medicine in Israel: consultation patterns of the Israeli population and attitudes of primary care physicians. Social Science and Medicine 44: 1341–1348

Burg MA, Hatch RL, Neims AH 1998 Lifetime use of alternative therapy: a study of Florida residents. Southern Medical Journal 91: 1126–1131

Eisenberg DM, Kessler RC et al 1993 Unconventional medicine in the United States: prevalence, costs and pattern use. New England Journal of Medicine 328: 246–252

Ernst E, Cassileth BR 1998 The prevalence of complementary/alternative medicine in cancer: a systematic review. Cancer 83: 777–782

Harris P, Rees R 2000 The prevalence of complementary and alternative medicine use among the general population: a systematic review of the literature. Complementary Therapies in Medicine 8: 88–96

Landmark Healthcare 1998 The Landmark Report on Public Perceptions of Alternative Care. Landmark Healthcare, Sacramento, USA

Linde K, Ramirez G et al 1996 St John's wort for depression – an overview and meta-analysis of randomised controlled trials. British Medical Journal 313: 253–258

Little C, Parsons T 2001 Herbal therapy for treating rheumatoid arthritis. Cochrane Database Syst Rev(1): CD002948

MacLennan AH, Wiilson DH, Taylor AW 1996 Prevalence and cost of alternative medicine in Australia. Lancet **347**: 569–573

Millar WJ 1997 Use of alternative health care practitioners by Canadians. Canadian Journal of Public Health **88**: 154–158

Paramore LC 1997 Use of alternative therapies: estimates from the 1994 Robert Wood Johnson Foundation National Access to Care Survey. Journal of Pain and Symptom Management **13**: 83–89

Thomas KJ, Fall M, Nicholl J, Williams B 1993 Methodological study to investigate the feasibility of conducting a population-based survey of the use of complementary health care. SCHARR, University of Sheffield, UK

Vaskilampi T, Merilainen P, Sinkkonen S 1993 The use of alternative treatments in the Finnish adult population. In: Lewith GT, Aldridge D (eds) Clinical research methodology for complementary therapies. Hodder and Stoughton, London

Verhoef MJ, Russell ML, Love EJ 1994 Alternative medicine use in rural Alberta. Canadian Journal of Public Health **85**: 308–309

Vernon H, McDermaid C et al 1999 Systematic review of randomized clinical trials of complementary/alternative therapies in the treatment of tension-type and cervicogenic headache. Complementary Therapies in Medicine **7**(3): 142–155

Yung B, Lewis M, Charny M, Farrow S 1988 Complementary medicine: some population-based data. Complementary Medicine Research **3**: 23–28

Collecting data

Sampling

11

WHY USE SAMPLING?

Sampling is used when it would be too impractical or logistically impossible to work with the entire population. A population in this case refers to all the cases that the researcher is interested in, whether they be people, events or objects. It could be all patients in a geographical area, all users of a particular service or all written policy guidelines within an organisation. This clearly presents practical problems when the population is very large or spread over a wide geographical area. Sampling is a way of working with subsets of the population to make the task more manageable. The selection process for sampling needs careful consideration and must be linked to the aims of the research. If the researcher expects the findings of the research to be generalisable to the entire population in question then the sample selected must be representative of the larger group. There are various sampling techniques for achieving this that fall under the heading of probability sampling.

TYPES OF SAMPLING

Systematic sampling

In this method every nth member of the population is included in the sample. Again this clearly requires a complete list of the population. For instance, in a population of 500 every 10th member on the list would be chosen for inclusion in the sample of 50. A crucial requirement for this form of sampling to be successful is that the ordering of the list is in no way related to the subject of the survey.

Quota sampling

The basic aim of quota sampling is to obtain adequate representation from the various subgroups of a population. Each subgroup is assigned a quota that the researcher will seek to fill. For example, it may be desirable to gather data from different age groups and a quota will be set for age groups 18–30, 31–45, 46–65 and 65+, so that the data are not gathered only from those who are most accessible or likely to participate in the research. While the aim is to gather a representative sample without randomisation, the process is subject to biases that probability sampling attempts to address.

Probability sampling

The essence of probability sampling is that each member of the population has an equal chance of being selected. There are various ways of achieving this.

RANDOM SAMPLING

In this method each member of the population has an equal chance of being selected into the sample. A requirement for using this method is a complete list of the population so that certain members are not excluded. This is called the sampling frame. Randomly choosing names from a hat is a simple example of this method. Obviously, if some names are not in the hat then they do not have a chance of being chosen. This is important because all those excluded may share common characteristics that make them different from the rest of the population. For instance, in seeking the opinions of drug users in an area only those whose names are kept on a register may be included. There may be drug users in an area that are not registered and therefore their opinions would be excluded.

STRATIFIED SAMPLING

Probability sampling is widely used in healthcare research to ensure all members of the population have an equal chance of being selected. However, in a non-homogeneous population minorities have a lesser chance of being represented. By dividing the population into different groups or strata along the lines of shared characteristics, e.g. age or gender, it is possible to ensure that each subgroup is represented. Once the population has been stratified, random sampling is used within each stratum. Proportionate sampling is where the numbers in the sample strata reflect the actual numbers in the population. For example, if 10% of users of a service are 80+ years of age, then 10% of the sample should be over 80. Disproportionate sampling is where more than the actual percentage in the population are included in the sample. This may be important where a small sample would be inadequate to represent the range of opinions or experiences of, say, the over-80s. Choosing the relevant categories for sampling depends upon the purpose of the study. Choices can be made as to which subgroups within the population might need to be differentiated. This process helps the researcher ensure accurate representation of the population under study. What is important is that stratification is carefully performed to ensure that the groupings are genuine.

CLUSTER SAMPLING

With this technique the population is divided into subgroups based on defined characteristics. These clusters are then chosen on a random basis and all the sub-population in the cluster is included within the sample (Fig. 11.1). This technique is useful when simple random sampling may generate a widely dispersed geographical sample, which could mean an interviewer having to track up and down the country. There is, however, a trade-off between convenience and a lack of precision. With cluster sampling it is difficult to ensure the sample is truly representative of the whole population.

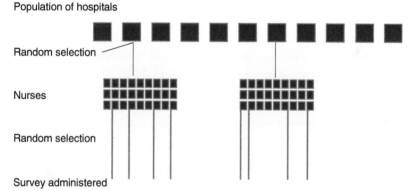

Figure 11.1   Cluster sampling.

MULTI-STAGE SAMPLING

This is taking samples from samples. An extension of cluster sampling, it similarly provides a means of generating a geographically concentrated sampling. For example, from a random sample of hospitals one might then take a random sample of nursing staff from each of the selected hospitals. This process can be iterated, with successive samples being drawn from the previous level, e.g. nurses with a postgraduate qualification in complementary therapies. The advantage of this is that the nurses who are finally surveyed will be grouped together in the selected hospitals (Box 11.1). The problem with cluster techniques is that one cannot be sure that the sample chosen does not differ in some significant way from the rest of the population and therefore the representativeness or external validity may be open to question. If the whole population is homogeneous in the characteristics being researched, then it could be expected that the selected sample would fairly represent the population as a whole. But to use our example of nurses, it may be that one of the unselected hospitals had a greater concentration of nurses with postgraduate qualifications in complementary therapies because hospital policy supported postgraduate training and gave scope for practice. None of these nurses would have any chance of being included in the sample.

Box 11.1   Multi-stage cluster sampling

- Population of all hospitals in a region – randomised
- Sub-population of nurses drawn from selected hospitals – randomised
- Nurses with postgraduate qualification in complementary therapies – randomised

---

SAMPLE SIZE

A question often asked is what size sample will I need? Unfortunately, no magic number can be given and the answer is not straightforward. It depends on a number of factors of which the researcher will have to weigh up the relative importance when deciding on sample size.

If the aim is to work with a sample that is representative of the whole population, then a larger sample is more likely to be representative than a small one. There are, however, diminishing returns and to avoid wasting valuable resources some calculation of the minimum size sample is required. The actual numbers depend on the type of study and the population concerned. If you intend to use inferential statistics, for instance in determining the effectiveness of an intervention, you need to know what the degree of expected change is from the intervention, as well as knowing the population characteristics. If the treatment effect is small (in relation to the control group or baseline), then you will need a fairly large sample to be able to determine with confidence that your findings were not a result of chance factors (see Ch. 8, Experiments and quasi-experiments). If the treatment effect is large (in relation to the control group or baseline), then the sample size can be reduced accordingly.

Resources are often a determining factor that limit sample size. When working with smaller samples the analysis must be kept simple. Each subdivision made in the data requires increased numbers to ensure that a representative sample is in the subdivision. Below a certain sample size, most forms of statistical analysis become meaningless. The opinion of a statistician can be extremely valuable at this stage to ensure that you have a clear idea of the numbers required in each subset.

Non-probability sampling

What defines non-probability sampling is that those included in the sample are not chosen on a random basis. Attempting to define a representative sample is not always desirable in case study and some qualitative designs. The researcher will purposively choose the sample, making judgements based on where the most valuable data are likely to be obtained. This contrasts sharply with probability sampling, where the researcher attempts to stand back and let chance factors determine who or what should be included in the sample.

PURPOSIVE SAMPLING

In purposive sampling the researcher uses knowledge of the population to locate the most useful informants. Of course, a process that does not exclude bias cannot claim representativeness, but in the research traditions that make use of purposive sampling representativeness is not what is aimed for. For instance, one could survey a random sample of healthcare workers in a hospital on the issues involved in integrating complementary therapies in a hospital setting. Alternatively, using purposive sampling, those individuals with experience of trying to integrate complementary therapies and those responsible at a policy level would be sought out, because their opinions would be informed and influential.

SNOWBALL SAMPLING

This kind of sample grows through individuals included in the initial sample nominating others who would be relevant for the research. These people are contacted in anticipation of including them in the sample. This process can be extended until all the relevant criteria for the sample are fulfilled. By using respondents with 'insider knowledge' the researcher builds the sample purposively. This approach can be useful where no sampling frame exists, i.e. when there is no complete list of the population in question (see below for an explanation of sampling frames). A disadvantage of this technique is that only members of a specific network will be included.

Theoretical sampling

The emphasis of this sampling technique, described by Glaser and Strauss (1967), is on the development of theory. As theories are generated from in-depth interviews about the topic being researched, the researcher attempts to locate respondents who can provide data that will expand and challenge the developing theory. This requires the researcher actively to seek out respondents of differing characteristics and experience. No attempt is made to randomly select the sample. Like 'extreme case' or 'rare element' samples, these are sought out because they contrast with the norm and their very different experience may shed new light on the phenomena in question.

Incidental or convenience sampling

This is sometimes used as a rough-and-ready way of building a survey sample, using the easiest and most convenient persons to act as respondents until the required sample size has been reached. This does not produce representative findings and is prone to all kinds of unspecified bias in who is included in the sample. Whilst such an approach may be helpful in piloting a survey or getting a feel for the issues, it forms a poor basis for generalisation and has none of the specificity of a purposively selected sample.

THE SAMPLING FRAME

This is a complete list of the population of interest. This might be based on geography, gender or any other determinant such as medical condition or users of a particular service. The list should be complete and up-to-date. There are commercial companies that sell lists of organisations or private individuals in a postal district. If the population of interest is of particular professionals, say osteopaths or occupational therapists, then the professional or regulatory bodies are sometimes willing to provide lists on computer disc or labels for a fee. If the population of interest is within an organisation, there may be lists of all employees, all patients with a particular condition, all complaints etc. The difficulty is in ensuring that the list is both complete and up-to-date and therefore a good basis for a representative sample. There may be members of a population who are not included on a list; for example, a list of hospital employees might not include self-employed contractors.

In summary, the sampling frame must be relevant for the subject, complete, up-to-date and precise, i.e. it excludes items not relevant to the research.

CONCLUSION

Obtaining truly representative samples can be very difficult or even impossible and investigating how practical it is to access your population of interest is a crucial piece of development work. An organisation may be unwilling to provide you with a list of employees or patients. It is important to try and negotiate access to such lists at a very early stage of the research. The use of inadequate sampling techniques is one of the most common problems in healthcare research. For an example of the difficulties that can occur when samples are not matched correctly in an observational study, see the discussion of the paper by Bagnel et al (1990), on p. 91 in Chapter 8, Experiments and quasi-experiments.

References

Bagnel F, Easton D et al 1990 Survival of patients with breast cancer attending Bristol Cancer Help Centre. Lancet **336**: 606–610
Glaser B, Strauss A 1967 The discovery of grounded theory. Aldine, Chicago

Interviews

INTRODUCTION

Interviews are a very useful and popular way of gathering research data. They are accessible, low tech and utilise basic conversation skills held by virtually everyone. They are highly flexible and adaptable and can be put to a wide variety of uses. In fact the majority of social science research is based on interview data such as that gathered in surveys, evaluations and ethnographic studies. It is, however, a misconception to think that interviews provide an easy option requiring little planning and forethought. As with every form of research, there are many issues that need to be carefully considered before undertaking the study. The first is whether interviews are the most suitable tool in answering your research question or whether questionnaires, observation or other methods of data collection might be more appropriate.

WHEN TO USE INTERVIEWS

Interviews can provide information on people's opinions, attitudes, beliefs and behaviours. The data can be used for descriptive, exploratory or explanatory studies. Simple factual information can be obtained through a highly structured interview, but using a self-report questionnaire may be a more efficient way of gathering such data, especially when the sample is large or geographically spread. When in-depth or complex information is required, interviews are able to provide data that are not easily obtained through any other means. You should consider whether your research requires the detailed information provided by interviews, and whether in-depth data from a small number of respondents are likely to be more useful than more superficial information from a larger sample of your research population.

Interviews are useful when the issues are complex or sensitive. Interviews can be flexible enough to take account of the linkages that the respondent makes to the subject. Most people will have felt the frustration of filling in a questionnaire that did not seem to have the category of response required and then scrawling in the margins or ticking between the boxes. Loosely structured interviews allow respondents to frame their answers in a way that makes sense to them and sets out the context of their response.

Interviews, like questionnaires, can only produce data on what respondents say they do. There is often a gap between observed behaviour and self-reporting. This does not mean the data are of no value but it does call for caution in interpretation.

TYPES OF INTERVIEW

The highly structured interview

In a highly structured interview the respondent is asked very specific pre-formulated questions set by the researcher. This form of interview is used in surveys, where small amounts of pre-coded data are collected through face-to-face or telephone interviews. The researcher will already have determined the categories of responses and the respondent supplies answers to a set of specific questions. The answers can then be scaled (from strongly disagree to strongly agree) or scored (0–10). This makes the data amenable to quantitative analysis where the scores of all the respondents can be added together to establish averages or to map out ranges of response. This has all the advantages and disadvantages described in Chapter 9, Surveys. A structured interview schedule will look very similar to a structured questionnaire but the interviewer writes the responses in. The face-to-face contact allows the interviewer to explain or clarify the questions. The reader should refer to Chapter 13, Questionnaires.

The qualitative interview

Although qualitative interviews can be highly structured, more typically they take advantage of the flexibility offered by the interview situation, from completely open-ended interviews, in which the conversation has only the loosest boundaries and the structure is defined by the respondent, to semi-structured interviews, where specific areas are identified by the researcher who will attempt to direct the interview to cover these areas.

Completely open-ended interviews may be useful when the boundaries of the topic are not clear or if you are interested in the links and connections that respondents make when exploring the topic area. The unstructured interview is the typical mode of collection in ethnographic studies, where the researcher is attempting to get an insider's viewpoint. A less-structured format can also be useful when the topic is sensitive and the interviewer can reorder or reword the questions to help put the respondent at ease.

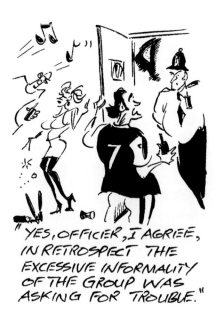

"YES, OFFICER, I AGREE, IN RETROSPECT THE EXCESSIVE INFORMALITY OF THE GROUP WAS ASKING FOR TROUBLE."

Formal or informal

In ethnographic work many of the interviews are informal, and the researcher becomes a participant observer in the activities of the research site. Two key issues that should be considered here are the ethics of interviewing and recording the interview data. It is important to have worked through the ethics of your research and addressed the question of informed consent (and gained the approval of the ethics committee responsible for your area). There is an argument that if an individual is to participate in the research by being interviewed, then that person's full informed consent should be sought. It may not be feasible, practical or desirable to have each and every person you converse with sign a consent form. The principles that no one should suffer as a result of the research and that individual identities should not be disclosed are sound and should be adhered to. Gaining consent for a formal interview is more straightforward and the normal requirement is that the respondent signs a consent form. The reader should refer to Chapter 4, Research ethics, for further discussion of these issues.

Face-to-face or telephone

Face-to-face interviews facilitate the development of rapport and allow response to non-verbal cues. This may be important when sensitive issues are being discussed. A disadvantage of face-to-face interviews is the effort required to set up the interview, including arranging a mutually convenient time and place as well as travelling to the interview. Telephone interviews are easier to arrange and the trade-offs between the two types of interview will need to be weighed up (see Ch. 9, Surveys).

RECORDING THE INTERVIEW

To gain useful data for analysis there will need to be some way of recording the interview. Memory is not especially reliable and is prone to selective recall. For informal interviews within an ethnographic study you may need to rely on field notes taken as soon as possible after the interview. Taking notes whilst being a participant observer may disturb the naturalness of the setting that you are trying to capture. This may mean absenting yourself from the setting to make notes in private (frequent bathroom visits are sometimes used by urban ethnographic researchers). Field notes will create a permanent record of your interpretation of what was said and can be referred back to at a later date. Such documents are clearly an interpretation rather than a record of fact that can be objectively verified. In a more formal interview setting you may be able to audio- or even video-record the interviews. If the information is sensitive, then respondents may be unwilling to divulge this with a recorder on. You will need to assess the feasibility of using a recording device within your research setting. Even if the information is not especially sensitive, having a recorder on will be disconcerting to many respondents. That said, if an audio-recorder is used unobtrusively, most people get beyond their initial hesitancy, and the advantage of having a hard recording of the data outweighs the initial disruption. There is very little justification for covert recording and you should always seek the explicit permission of the interviewee prior to commencing the recording.

It is absolutely crucial that your equipment is well prepared before the interview. This means having a good power supply (and spare batteries) and tape of sufficient length so that you do not have to fiddle with the recorder to change tapes in the middle of an interview. Consider using one of the newer-generation minidisc recorders which can allow longer recording times and the possibility of storage on your computer. You should be familiar enough with the recorder to know how to place it unobtrusively and get sufficient sound/visual reproduction for transcribing later.

Double check your recording equipment before using it and always carry spare batteries and tapes!

It is helpful to keep notes even when you record the interview. These notes can record contextual information and the researcher's impressions about the situation. There are also things that a tape recorder cannot capture, such as non-verbal communication, making interview notes invaluable during analysis. You should try to record these notes during or as soon as practicable after the interview, while your memory of the event is still fresh.

INTERVIEWER SKILLS

The skills of an individual interviewer can have a determining effect on the content of an interview. The personal characteristics of the interviewer, the rapport developed with the respondent, and the type and ordering of questions can all influence what people will say in an interview.

Rapport

Successful interviews are based on the development of trust and rapport. Respondents need to feel that they are being understood and that what they have to say is being valued. This does not mean the interviewer has an obligation to agree with the respondent's opinions, but an attitude of respect will usually facilitate the interview process.

Interviewer effect

There are various personal characteristics of the interviewer that may influence what a respondent will say in an interview. These include gender, age, ethnicity and social status. How these will impact on the interview will depend to some extent on the topic being explored. An interview on race relations or immigration policy might have a very different flow or even produce quite different data depending upon the ethnicities of the interviewer and the respondent. Embarrassment or defensiveness may inhibit honest responses. There is a well-recognised tendency for respondents to give answers they believe will meet the expectations of the interviewer.

Researchers should be aware that how they present themselves can influence the data that are collected. Whilst essential characteristics of the interviewer such as age, gender and ethnicity are not readily changed or disguised, some characteristics can be modified in ways that may influence the data that are collected. Researchers' attitudes to interview topics and their verbal and non-verbal responses through the interview are likely to influence what the respondents have to say.

The general advice is for interviewers to remain neutral or non-committal to the statements made, in an attempt to minimise their impact and avoid biasing the responses. This fits with the idea of a detached and neutral researcher whose main function is to draw out data from respondents with minimal impact.

One argument against this cool detachment is that this attitude will also have its influence on what respondents say. The responses that people give are always context bound. If the context of the interview is one in which an outsider (the interviewer, whose own attitudes and beliefs are concealed in a bid for neutrality) has come in to take away information that will be used for the interviewer's own purposes, then the responses are likely to be framed very differently to responses to an interviewer whose enthusiasm and commitment for a particular position is clearly expressed.

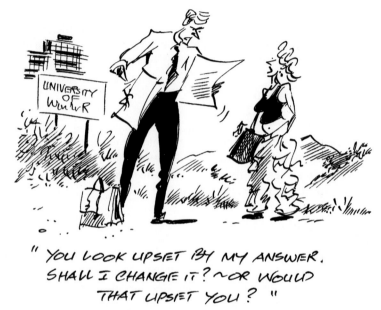

" YOU LOOK UPSET BY MY ANSWER.
SHALL I CHANGE IT? ~OR WOULD
THAT UPSET YOU? "

A note of caution: a passionate and engaged approach to interviewing may be appropriate when the aim of the research is to facilitate and empower, as is typical in action research projects. It is more likely to be seen as bad practice and a source of bias in most other traditions of research. You need to consider carefully the aims of the research and the audience your research is intended for, e.g. university examiners, journal editors, policy makers or funders of community development projects.

Framing the questions

Both the type of questions asked and the ordering of those questions will influence the responses given. In a formal interview you should give some consideration to the ordering of questions. It is usual to start with 'warm up' questions to put the respondent at ease. Straightforward factual questions that are easily answered should precede more complex or demanding questions. You should ensure that the questions are framed simply and unambiguously. Many of the considerations in designing questionnaires also apply to interviewing and you should review the issues discussed in Chapter 13, Questionnaires, when preparing your interview schedules.

The key points to remember when you are framing questions are listed in Box 12.1.

Box 12.1   Key paints when preparing questions

- Keep the questions simple and short
- Avoid double-barrelled questions (where questions are joined together)
- Don't use jargon unless necessary
- Avoid leading questions

The interviewer is doing much more than acting as a scribe. While identifying the main points being stated, the interviewer also attempts to read between the lines to grasp the underlying logic of the statements and, sometimes more importantly, what is not being said. It may be appropriate to seek clarification on ambiguities and inconsistencies later on in the interview. Not that we should expect everything people say to be absolutely consistent; it may be the work of our analysis later on to account for these ambiguities and inconsistencies. We should bear in mind that the context of a question may alter the response to the same question half an hour later, as different priorities come into the foreground.

Effective interviewers will use conversational devices to progress the interview. These are described in the methodology literature as probes, prompts and checks — words probably best left out of actual interviews because of their invasive connotations (see Box 12.2). These devices should be applied with subtlety and sensitivity as part of the natural conversational flow of the

---

Box 12.2   Probes, prompts and checks

Probes

A probe is a follow-up question inviting interviewees to clarify or give more detail about their response. Questions asking for an example or what, how, why and when are ways of encouraging the respondent to go deeper into a particular area.

Prompts

The judicious use of silence is one of the best ways to prompt the respondent to elaborate, along with non-verbal cues such as nodding the head. An encouraging 'uh-huh' can indicate to respondents that what they are saying is relevant and that they should continue.

Checks

As part of the interview dialogue, interviewers are able to check they have got an accurate understanding of what was said. This may be done by asking respondents to repeat what they have said or by presenting a summary for confirmation or correction. These summaries can also be used to bring closure to particular areas being discussed and to move the interview along.

---

interview. Try not to make respondents feel inarticulate or that what they have said is inadequate; rather, you should convey that it is the interviewer who has failed to understand fully what was meant and who needs clarification.

Asking questions

How questions are worded should be carefully considered. Although it is possible to clarify questions for respondents, you should attempt to be as clear as possible in the first instance. Chapter 13, Questionnaires, explores this more fully but it is worth highlighting here some key points (Box 12.3).

Box 12.3 Key points in asking questions

- Keep the questions short, clear and simple
- The style of the questions should be appropriate to the respondents
- Ask one question at a time — avoid double-barrelled questions
- Avoid dichotomous questions that invite simple yes/no answers
- Ask genuinely open-ended questions that invite respondents to choose to answer in their own terms
- Avoid presuppositions in the questions
- Avoid leading questions
- Avoid vague questions
- Consider carefully the type of question you intend to ask and the level of response you are seeking:
  - factual information
  - personal experience or behaviours
  - opinions and values
  - feeling questions

TRANSCRIBING INTERVIEWS

Transcribing audio tapes is not as straightforward as it might seem. The actual task of transcribing is very time-consuming and you can reckon on several hours transcribing for every hour of tape. Just how long it takes will depend on whether you have access to transcribing equipment, how clear the recording is, and your own typing speed. Transcribing machines provide a foot-operated rewind, play and stop button to use while you are typing and this speeds up the task considerably. If the recordings are not very clear you will probably need to rewind and listen again to what was said. When things are not entirely clear you will have to make a judgement about whether to scrap that piece of data or include it in an incomplete form.

It is a fact that many people do not speak in clear logical sentences and rely on intonation, body language and context to make themselves understood. If this is not immediately obvious, it will be when you attempt to transcribe the interviews. The problem will be compounded if the recording is of a group interview, where people talk over the top of each other. The researcher will need to edit the work sufficiently so that it becomes intelligible on the written page. Intonations and body language can change the meaning of words, but these are not easily conveyed in writing. When these intonations, accents or body language are central to the meaning of what is being said, the researcher should try and indicate this by the use of bracketed comments or separate field notes which set out some of the contextual factors. In traditions such as discourse analysis, a range of standard codes have been developed to record this extralinguistic information. There is an inevitable editorial process that the researcher engages in while transcribing, which means that the truth value of the data is not beyond question. A useful check on the accuracy of the transcript is to have respondents review it. Though they may not remember if the transcript is word-for-word correct, they will be able to confirm the accuracy of facts and whether they stand by the feelings or opinions expressed at the time of interview.

ANALYSIS OF INTERVIEWS

How you will analyse your interview data needs to be thought about at the design stage of the research, not when you have the interview transcripts in front of you. There needs to be congruence between the guiding research question and your method of analysis. Your choice of analytic method will depend upon why the interviews were conducted. If you are interested in the strategies people use to cope with chronic back pain, then a narrative approach to analysis may be appropriate. If, on the other hand, you want to describe the range of self-help behaviours used by people with chronic back pain, then a categorising methodology will be more appropriate. The research question will guide your choice of method. The research question and the approach to analysis will also determine the kinds of questions you should be asking in the interview. See Section 4 for further explanation of the range of analytic approaches.

VALIDITY

What is said in an interview situation cannot be taken at face value. The responses must be seen as a product of the interview situation. The degree of honesty will vary. It goes beyond simply whether people are telling the truth: by whom, how, where and why the interviews are conducted will have a determining effect on what people say. Far from being recordings of self-evident truths, interviews require a degree of interpretation in even the simplest situations and topics. The extent to which people mean what they say and say what they mean, as well as the filters and interpretative framework used by the researcher, need to be weighed up when making validity judgements about interview research. The steps the researcher has taken to check the validity and the interpretation of the data should be made explicit. This is so that readers of research reports are able to judge for themselves how far the researchers have gone to establish the validity of their work.

ADVANTAGES

✔ A flexible research tool that can be applied in a wide range of situations with simple equipment

✔ Able to provide in-depth accounts

✔ Able to capture the respondent's perspective

✔ Good response rate compared to postal questionnaires

✔ Sampling strategy can be adjusted along the way according to demand. With postal questionnaires it may not be clear until the analysis phase whether all the important subgroups of the population have been represented

DISADVANTAGES

✘ Resource intensive: interviewing, transcribing and analysis are time-consuming, as is travelling to the interviews when the respondents are geographically spread out

✘ The responses people give are influenced by the context in which the interview takes place. The interviewer–respondent relationship, the place and timing and many other variables can influence what people say and how they say it. This calls into question the reliability of the data

✘ Informal, unstructured and semi-structured interviews produce non-standardised data, making analysis very open to interpretation. Demonstrating that the inferences made from the data are valid is made more complex by this fact

Further reading

Kvale S 1996 Interviews: an introduction to qualitative research interviewing. Sage, Thousand Oak

Questionnaires

13

INTRODUCTION

Everyone is familiar with filling in questionnaires of one sort or another. They are, perhaps, the most widely used research tool and the bedrock of survey research. In essence, a questionnaire is a list of questions for the purpose of research. Questionnaires can be used to gather data on what people think, feel and believe as well as more factual details. The factual information might include basic information such as age and gender, or particular activities and behaviours such as people's smoking or exercise habits. The responses can be given in a variety of formats and may be self-administered or filled in by an interviewer.

Questionnaires are an extremely useful tool when you require information from a large number of people and the information needed is fairly straightforward. When the responses to those questions can be standardised, it makes the process of analysing a large data set relatively simple.

PLANNING

The key to successfully developing and using a questionnaire lies in planning and organisation. There is a sequence of steps that you will need to follow to produce a credible questionnaire. Because at its most basic the method is nothing more than a list of questions, it is too easy to underestimate the time required to develop, administer and analyse successfully the responses to a questionnaire. You will need to allocate time for the following steps:

- *Design*: you need to define specifically the areas you want the questionnaire to address. Spend some time getting to know the crucial issues. It can help to conduct several in-depth interviews with those in the know, such as patients or professionals with first-hand knowledge of the field of interest. From these discussions you should draw up a list of possible questions. The key issues and the information you require from respondents should be kept in the foreground. The questions formulated in relation to these issues must be clear and concise. The questions then need to be ordered and a suitable layout created. The design stage is elaborated later in this chapter, but having developed a draft questionnaire you then need to allow sufficient time for the following steps.
- *Piloting*: having established the key issues and formulated an initial set of questions, you should pre-pilot them on colleagues to see whether they make sense to others and whether the answers provided relate to the intended topic. You should then test the questionnaire for ease of administration and response with a subgroup of the population you are interested in. However clear a question may appear to you, others may interpret this differently.
- *Corrections*: should be made on the basis of feedback and the responses from the pre-pilot and pilot questionnaires.
- *Production*: once you have created a final draft of the questionnaire, you will need to allow time for production of copies including identification numbers for each questionnaire (be aware that identification numbers may clash with a requirement for anonymity).
- *Distribution*: whether this is by post or face-to-face, you should calculate the time required for this.
- *Response time*: this will vary with the population concerned, but by 2 or 3 weeks the majority of those intending to respond will have done so.
- *Follow-up of non-respondents*: depending on the level of response received, you may decide to send a repeat mailing to those who have not replied. A judgement has to be made on the value of the extra time and effort required for this, as the response rate for follow-ups is typically low.
- *Collation and checking of the data*: for accuracy and completeness in responses.
- *Analysis*: pre-coded responses are fairly straightforward compared to the categorising of open responses. You need to be clear from the outset what kind of statistical tests you intend to apply to the data. Interpreting the significance of qualitative data is demanding, and you will probably need to 'eat, breathe and sleep with the data' for some time.
- *Presentation of results*: this may be through narrative alone or with tables and diagrams. Ensure you allow time for learning how to use any unfamiliar software to help you with the presentation.

These steps are summarised in Box 13.1.

Box 13.1   Steps in developing and using a questionnaire

- Designing questionnaire
- Piloting questionnaire
- Corrections based on pilot
- Production of questionnaire
- Distribution
- Response time
- Follow-up of non-respondents
- Collation and preparation of data
- Analysis
- Presentation of results

COSTS AND RESOURCES

You will need to calculate for the resources required to develop and carry through your questionnaire research. If you have worked through the planning stages above, you should have some idea of the time scale. In terms of how many hours you will need to allocate, it is worth remembering that in research things always take much longer than expected.

Obvious costs are the production and posting of the questionnaires. You will need to consider the cost of supplying stamped addressed envelopes and the cost of follow-up of non-respondents. Desktop publishing software may be required to produce a high-quality questionnaire. You will need access to the software and time to develop skilful use. If you intend to have this done professionally, the costs for this will need to be built in. Likewise for data analysis software; you will need to consider access and development of skills or getting outside help.

CONSTRUCTING THE QUESTIONNAIRE

Background information

A covering letter or the front page of each questionnaire should contain background information about the research and the questionnaire. This should include:

- Who is conducting the research: if it is under the auspices of an institution or organisation, this should be stated. It is often helpful to include a named researcher who can be contacted should there be any queries about the research
- Why the research is being undertaken: the focus of the questionnaire as well as the potential beneficiaries

- What is required: the amount of time a respondent will need to spend to complete the questionnaire and the kind of information you would like them to provide
- What can be expected: an express promise to respect confidentiality or anonymity (depending on the nature of the research)
- Where to return the completed questionnaire: clear instructions should be given on the cover page as well as at the end of the questionnaire
- Thanks for co-operation and participation.

Identifying subject areas

The researcher needs to reflect very carefully on the central research question. This should be broken down into distinct subject areas or topics for which specific questions can then be formulated for inclusion in the questionnaire. You need to clarify the distinctions between the subject areas or topics, so that the questions you formulate are unambiguously related to that specific area. This is to ensure that the answers are oriented towards exactly that topic and not a related but different topic.

Wording the questions

It takes a lot of effort and refining to come up with a list of good questions. As well as ensuring that the questions are clearly linked to the subject area, it is critical that the researcher ensures that respondents are not confused by the questions. To this end:

- The vocabulary should match the reading skills and knowledge base of the population of respondents.
- The questions should be easily understood and unambiguous.
- Technical jargon should be kept to a minimum.
- Short simple sentences are preferable to long complex ones.
- Avoid double-barrelled questions – i.e. asking more than one question at a time, e.g. Do you currently work more than 50 hours a week and are you satisfied with this? This example should be broken down into two separate questions.
- Avoid vague questions – be specific and concrete.
- Avoid leading questions.
- Avoid double negatives.

You should consider carefully the type of question you intend to ask and the level of response you are seeking:

- Factual information
- Personal experience or behaviours
- Opinions and values
- Feeling questions.

Some key points to help you in wording your questions are given in Box 13.2.

Box 13.2   Key points to remember in wording the questions

- Keep the questions short, clear and simple.
- The style of the questions should be appropriate to the respondents.
- Ask one question at a time – avoid double-barrelled questions.
- Avoid dichotomous questions that invite simple yes–no answers (unless, of course, you want a yes–no answer).
- Ask genuinely open-ended questions that invite respondents to choose to answer in their own terms.
- Avoid presuppositions in the questions.
- Avoid leading questions.
- Avoid vague questions.

CLOSED QUESTIONS

Closed questions restrict the choice of available responses. Pre-set answers usually require less effort from respondents than a blank space, and ease of completing is likely to have a positive effect on response rates. They also make analysis simpler as the range of responses is already known and pre-coded. However, the available choices should cover the range of responses likely to be given. This requires substantial effort in the design phase, with appropriate piloting of the questionnaire, perhaps starting with open questions to gauge the range of responses. Careful piloting of open questions can lead to the development of useful closed questions. When the range of possible responses cannot be narrowed, you may require an 'other' (please specify) category. Closed answer questions are most effective when the topic being covered is fairly straightforward. The subtlety and nuance of response that is possible in open questions is lost, but the trade-off is easily categorised data (see Box 13.3). There are various kinds of closed response questions and examples of these can be seen in Box 13.4, from the simplest agreement scale to a more complex five point 'Likert scale'. Each of the stages of agreement/disagreement is assigned a score and, where appropriate, this can be calculated to provide an overall score.

Box 13.3   Closed questions

- Restrict responses
- Allow less subtlety and nuance than open questions, but are
- Easy to respond to
- Simple to analyse as responses are pre-coded
- Appropriate when the topic is fairly straightforward

Box 13.4   Types of closed questions

Agree/Disagree (bipolar or 5 point Likert)

Please indicate your response to the following questions

Acupuncture should be widely available on the NHS

a) Bipolar

Agree   disagree

b) Likert scale

Strongly agree   agree   neutral   disagree   strongly disagree

Yes/No

Have you personally used any complementary therapies in the last year?

List of options

Choose one of the following options
Where would you prefer to see an acupuncturist?

1. in their private consulting rooms
2. in a local GP surgery
3. in a local hospital
4. in your own home

Rank order

From the following list please rank the services you would most like to see available within your local GP surgery. 1 indicates your strongest preference 2 the second strongest and so on until 5 indicates your least strong preference.
Acupuncture __ Chiropody__Dietician__Fitness instructor__ Osteopathy __

Rating scale

How significant an influence is the following on your own health?

	not significant			very significant	
Diet	1	2	3	4	5
Exercise	1	2	3	4	5
Exposure to environmental pollutants	1	2	3	4	5
Daily hassles	1	2	3	4	5
Your ability to relax and unwind	1	2	3	4	5
Medical interventions	1	2	3	4	5
Your relationships with other people	1	2	3	4	5

Semantic differential

Regular physical exercise is:

Difficult to make time for	1	2	3	4	5	easy to make time for
Not worth the effort	1	2	3	4	5	worth the effort
Likely to lead to injury	1	2	3	4	5	unlikely to lead to injury
Boring	1	2	3	4	5	interesting
Important for health	1	2	3	4	5	unimportant for health

OPEN QUESTIONS

An open question allows respondents to answer in whatever way makes sense to them. It is up to the respondents to choose the words they will use and the length of their responses. This is advantageous when the range of possible responses to a given question is unknown. It is also useful in the design phase to pilot the topic areas with open questions. The data will allow you to refine your choice of responses should you wish to develop a closed question. Because the responses are not predetermined, analysis is more complex but the richness in detail and nuance may compensate for lack of standardisation.

Ordering the questions

The ordering of questions can influence how or even whether people will respond to a questionnaire. You should identify the topics or sub-topics that are to be covered in the questionnaire and choose a running order for the topics. The numbering system should guide the respondent through the topic areas. It's usually best to ask people what they do before you ask what they believe or feel. Such factual questions are more straightforward to answer or abstract and can help orient the respondent to more general issues. The answers that respondents give at the beginning of an interview will strongly influence how they answer later questions.

RESPONSE RATE

A number of factors will influence the response rate to questionnaires. Time is an important factor. Busy working people will not have the same free time as those who are retired. Interest in the topic will also have a determining effect. It is up to you as the researcher to convince potential respondents why they should spend their valuable time in completing your questionnaire. Whether through a covering letter or face-to-face contact, the researcher will need to explain the relevance of the research to the respondents. The researcher may be able to highlight how the research will benefit respondents. Sometimes inducements are offered, such as entering respondents into a prize draw. If this is considered an option, the researcher will need to demonstrate that any inducements are not going to bias the responses. Questions that are seen as intrusive or insensitive are not likely to hold the goodwill of potential respondents and may be more than enough reason for them to put the questionnaire aside.

How easy a questionnaire appears to be to complete will also have a determining effect on response rates. A questionnaire that looks complex and time-consuming may put off potential respondents. Clarity and simplicity should be aimed for in the presentation and in the questions asked. Any instructions on filling in the questionnaire or what to do once it has been completed should also be simple and direct. It is good practice to give such

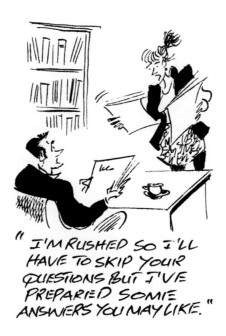

" I'M RUSHED SO I'LL
HAVE TO SKIP YOUR
QUESTIONS BUT I'VE
PREPARED SOME
ANSWERS YOU MAY LIKE. "

instructions on the covering letter as well as at the end of the questionnaire. With a bit of luck respondents will follow through with those instructions as soon as they have completed the questionnaire.

CODING THE RESPONSES

Closed response questions make the process of coding very straightforward and computer software packages such as Statistical Package for Social Scientists (SPSS) can help in the organisation of this. Each possible response is given a numerical value by the coder which is placed in a coding box in a narrow column down the right-hand side of the questionnaire. This allows the numbers to be efficiently transferred onto a computer file for processing (see Table 13.1).

The coding of open questions is more complicated as each response will have to be carefully read and allocated a place within a coding schema. At its simplest, the researcher will devise a scheme of possible response categories to each question and allocate each written statement accordingly. The approach to analysis will determine what kind of coding is required and various distinctive traditions of qualitative data analysis have evolved. Computer software packages can assist in coding and analysis and their utility will be discussed in Chapter 16, Analysing qualitative data.

Table 13.1 Coding responses		
Example question	**Answer**	**Coding numbers**
Question 1		
Do you smoke?	yes/no	__ (1 for yes, 2 for no)
Question 2		
How much do you smoke?		
Up to 5 per day	☐	__ (coded as 1)
Between 6 and 10 per day	☐	__ (coded as 2)
Between 11 and 20 per day	☐	__ (coded as 3)
Between 21 and 30 per day	☐	__ (coded as 4)
Between 31 and 40 per day	☐	__ (coded as 5)
More than 40 per day	☐	__ (coded as 6)

USING ESTABLISHED QUESTIONNAIRES

There are many tried and tested questionnaires on specific subject areas, such as general wellbeing and a wide range of specific diseases (Bowling 1991, 1995). The advantage of using such instruments is that they have usually been scrutinised and tested for their validity and reliability in relation to the topic area they cover. There is also the advantage of being able to compare the findings of your research to other studies using the same instrument, thus adding to the body of knowledge in your field.

The main disadvantage is that the focus of the instrument may be different from the questions that are driving your research. There is always the option of altering the focus of your study or of drawing on parts of the questionnaire that fit your own research. If you do wish to use an established questionnaire, then you need to check whether there are restricted licensing rights. In some cases the copyright rests with the authors who originated the instrument (tracked down through the address in the publication), and in other cases the licensing rights are owned by commercial companies. There may be restrictions on who the instruments will be supplied to, such as health researchers, and commercial companies will charge for use of the instrument. However, they will then normally provide the required number of copies of the questionnaire plus any scoring devices. If you use an established questionnaire you should, of course, cite this in any report you create. Examples of questionnaires, such as the Chiropratic revised Oswestry pain questionnaire, MYMOP and SF-36, can be seen in Chapter 8, Experiments and quasi-experiments.

ADVANTAGES

✔ Questionnaires are within the scope of most project researchers to devise, administer and analyse

✔ They are a straightforward way to find out what people think, feel, believe and do

✔ They are adaptable and may be used in a wide variety of settings

✔ It is relatively easy to gather large amounts of data. Once the development work has been done, data collection can be increased through postal distribution

✔ Relatively low costs. Although the cost of postage increases with wider distribution, the time and money spent in conducting face-to-face or even telephone interviews make postal questionnaires an economical option

✔ Data coding and analysis is greatly simplified when a closed answer format is used

DISADVANTAGES

✘ Short and simple questionnaires have the highest response rates but their brevity and simplicity may lead to oversimplification if the issues are complex. Longer and more detailed questionnaires may allow for a deeper analysis but a low response rate may lead to findings that are not truly representative of the study population

✘ Questionnaires have an extremely variable response rate, depending on factors such as the topic, study population and the quality and distribution method of the questionnaire. When the response rate is low it is extremely difficult to judge whether the data that are gathered accurately reflect the population as a whole or just the subset who were willing to respond to the questionnaire

✘ The accuracy of the responses to questionnaires, whether due to misinterpreting the questions or a lack of concern about providing accurate answers, can not be checked out. The researcher has no way of picking up clues and checking out the responses as they might in a face-to-face interview

References

Bowling A 1991 Measuring health: a review of quality of life measurement scales. Open University Press, Buckingham

Bowling A 1995 Measuring disease: a review of disease specific quality of life measurement scales. Open University Press, Buckingham

Further reading

Oppenheim A 2000 Questionnaire design, interviewing and attitude measurement. Continuum International Publishing Group, New York

Observations

14

INTRODUCTION

Using our own eyes is a fundamental way of knowing about the world. Whether we are interested in people and their activities, structures or processes, observation is a key method in research. It provides direct evidence rather than relying upon what people say. There is often a significant gap between what people say they do and what they actually do, and this gap is not necessarily intentional deceit. It is just that memory is not always a reliable guide to precise details and has a selective uptake and recall capacity. Observational methods in the broadest sense do not rely exclusively on visual data but include other direct sense data, such as smell or even touch. Observations can take place in highly controlled conditions, such as the laboratory, or out in the real world. Whilst there are some shared concerns about the reliability and validity of observations in both settings, this chapter will focus on observation that takes place out in the field. Observational methods can be complementary to other forms of data collection such as interviews, questionnaires or documents, providing either supportive or primary data.

STRUCTURED AND PARTICIPANT OBSERVATION

There are two main traditions that have influenced observational methods theory. The first is from social psychology. It takes many of the methods and assumptions of scientific laboratory work and applies them to fieldwork. It begins with framing a testable hypothesis. Using highly structured coding schedules with explicit coding criteria, observational data are collected that can be used to confirm or refute the research hypothesis. The emphasis on formal procedures is to manage observational bias and create a reproducible methodology (Croll 1986).

The second tradition has its origins in the social science of anthropology, which is the study of cultures. It attempts to understand those cultures by gaining an insider's view. The methodology developed for this is known as participant observation. Rather than beginning the observation with a fixed hypothesis and structured coding schedule, researchers immerse themselves within the daily goings on of the research site with a minimum of formality and structure, so as to observe how the culture operates from an insider's viewpoint (Lofland & Lofland 1995). The method of reporting these observations is typically in the form of a narrative rather than as a quantified set of results.

Key points of differences between structured and participant observation are given in Table 14.1.

Table 14.1   Key differences between structured and participant observation

Structured observation	Participant observation
Origins in psychology	Origins in anthropology
Testing a hypothesis	Understanding a culture through categories used within the culture
Use of coding schemes	
Highly structured observations	Relatively unstructured observations
Formal strategy	Informal strategy
Hypothesis confirmed or refuted	Develops narrative account
Develops an *etic* perspective	Develops an *emic* perspective

For explanatory purposes it is useful to describe these two traditions as polar opposites, but aspects of each tradition are frequently combined. In fact, it is typical for a highly structured coding scheme to be based on a period of unstructured observation, and equally participant observers may need to explicitly count and record activities and events to ensure that their interpretations are grounded in empirical observations.

DEVELOPING AN *EMIC* OR *ETIC* PERSPECTIVE

The *etic* perspective

These different methods of observation were developed in response to the questions and concerns of the respective disciplines. Early work in psychology highlighted the way in which human perception and memory could be influenced by the observers' expectations and past experience. The structured approach to observation standardises what is to be observed and how it is recorded, thereby minimising the degree of variation that can exist between observers. A high degree of inter-observer reliability provides evidence that the data collection has not been skewed by an individual observer's bias, and that the results may be considered to be objective. The *etic* perspective draws on the assumptions and categories of science rather than on how the observed make sense of their world. The *etic* perspective is typically adopted when using the structured approach.

The *emic* perspective

The concerns of anthropology have been to understand culture by learning about how insiders construct and perceive their world. To do this it is necessary to learn the ordering categories used within the specific culture. This generally requires a prolonged engagement and a willingness to learn by participating in the day-to-day activities that are given shape by the ordering categories. Working with a pre-set hypothesis and observation schedule will not help the researcher to understand how insiders view and order their own world — the *emic* perspective. The *emic* perspective is typically adopted when using participant observation.

STRUCTURED OBSERVATION

To address some of the problematic issues of selective perception and recall, the techniques of observation and recording are standardised. Coding schemes are developed that can range from simple checklists to complex multi-category schemes (Croll 1986). The basic concepts and categories are predefined according to the research hypothesis. The measures used by the observers should have a high degree of reliability, so that if more than one observer were to be positioned in practically the same place at the same time there would be a high degree of correlation between what the observers recorded (checked through a simple statistic known as percentage agreement). This may sound obvious, but if the criteria used for recording are not made explicit some of the observations may be viewed ambiguously and categorised differently. There are a number of rules for minimising this ambiguity, which are listed in Box 14.1.

Box 14.1   Defining the categories

- The categories for recording observations must be explicitly defined.
- The categories should be distinct and not overlapping, with clear boundaries as to whether an observation belongs in a particular category or not.
- The categories should be based on obvious behaviours that require minimal interpretation as to their meaning.
- Categorising the behaviour should not be highly dependent on the context of the behaviour, and therefore open to ambiguity.
- The observation should be easy to record.
- The observation schedule should comprehensively cover relevant observations.

Sampling

It is important to decide when, where and how the observations will take place.

TIMING

The timing of the observations should be designed to get a representative sample of the behaviours and activities under observation. Depending on the circumstances, the timings could be for 15 minutes every hour or in 1 hour blocks. Longer observations are not always better and may be too time intensive, without capturing the full range of behaviours that occur over a day, a week or whatever time period is relevant to the project.

LOCATION

How and where observers locate themselves can certainly influence the quality of the observations. Positioning yourself in a front row seat may provide a good vantage point for the action, but you need to remember that having a researcher with a clipboard ticking off observations may influence the behaviour of the observed. It may be better to locate yourself a bit more discreetly, providing you can still maintain an effective vantage given the focus of the research. Some locations are relatively easy to blend into. Students making notes in a university library are unlikely to change the behaviour of others in the library, as they do not look out of place. If, on the other hand, you enter a hospital ward (assuming

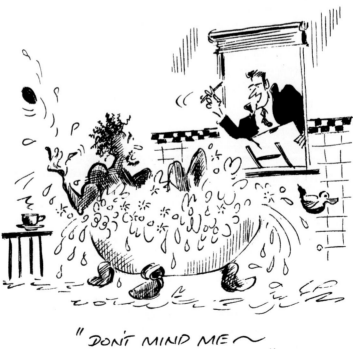

" DON'T MIND ME ~
I'M A RESEARCHER. "

you had permission to do so) and position yourself near the nursing station with clipboard in hand, it is unlikely that your presence will go unnoticed (with the consequence that behaviour around you will change as a result of your presence). When observing you should try to position yourself as unobtrusively as possible. How you achieve this may depend on the negotiations made when gaining access to the research site. Being unobtrusive is sometimes best achieved by behaving as a participant who is part of the everyday activity, rather than being an extremely big fly on the wall.

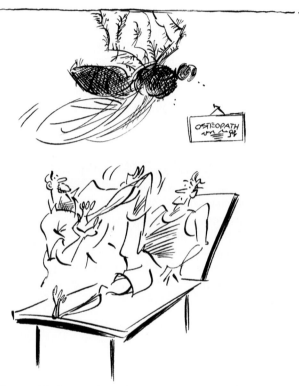

It is often said that with prolonged exposure people begin to take for granted a new presence, and many researchers report that, after an initial uneasiness about being observed, people seem to just get on with their daily activity. This is, of course, dependent upon what activities are being observed and what significance they have for the observed.

Keeping a record of contextual factors

Although the focus is on systematic recording of observations using standard categories, maintaining a record of any events or contextual factors can help to explain the observed behaviours. Relying exclusively on structured observational data may lead to an over-simplistic analysis, as the meaning of specific observations may only be revealed when seen in the context in which the events occurred. The record of contextual factors should be logged in relation to a specific set of observations.

PARTICIPANT OBSERVATION

Participant observation is contrasted to structured observation, although the dimensions of structure and participation are not mutually exclusive. It is possible to position yourself as a participant and collect structured data, and equally as a non-participant detached observer to collect unstructured observations.

Participant observation emphasises the collection of detailed, nuanced data that explain some of the complexity of the observed social world. By sharing in the world of the observed as a participant, the observer learns about the categories that insiders use to order and understand and function in their world.

Because of the mass of data surrounding the researcher you will need to decide what to attend to and record, and what to ignore. The conceptual framework and research focus will help define the relevant categories. Box 14.2, based on the categories of Spradley (1980), is a guide.

Box 14.2   Categorising your observation

- People and their behaviours – roles, social activities, tasks, specific actions, communications, conversations, interactions
- Environment – physical space, objects
- Events and meetings – routine, ritual, extraordinary
- Chronology – the temporal sequence of events and interactions, frequencies and durations of behaviours and events
- Maps – layout of site and people present.

From the early days of anthropology there has been the injunction to suspend preconceptions about what is observed and simply to immerse yourself in the situation, to learn to see the world as the insider does. Suspending all preconceptions is easier said than done, but the immersion needs to be sufficient so that you have really grasped the categories through which insiders make sense of their world. Although prolonged engagement can bring insiders' knowledge, there is also the danger of going native, i.e. an over-identification with the group being studied. As a researcher you have to hold both your own perspective (including the research questions and conceptual framework that initiated the study) and the perspective of the insider.

Recording observations

You should record what you see and hear in concrete terms. That means detailing the behaviours and words as they occurred, without jumping to an interpretation of their meaning. It is not always easy to maintain ongoing records as a participant. You need to be resourceful and discreet about your note taking, to avoid bringing unwanted attention to the fact that you are recording your observations. Frequent bathroom breaks or similar may be needed, to scribble up notes or speak into a dictaphone. Using shorthand or abbreviations for recurrent observations can be a great help. Covertly recording conversations raises ethical issues about informed consent, and in most instances would not be considered acceptable to an ethics committee assessing your research proposal (see Ch. 4, Research ethics).

At the end of an observation session your notes need to be written up in full, recording in detail everything that was observed. This should be as soon as possible after the event since recall becomes increasingly selective as past events recede. You should also record separately your own feelings and interpretations of the observations. This is the beginning of the analytic process. The categories for future observations are based on your interpretation of earlier observations. This is known as inductive analysis (see Ch. 16, Analysing qualitative data).

ADVANTAGES

✔ Observations do not rely on what people say they do, but examine what takes place in practice

✔ Observation requires minimal instrumentation; a pen and paper often suffice, with a schedule for systematic observations

✔ Insight gained about the workings of the observation site. By virtue of being on site, it is possible to gain an understanding of complex interactions and processes

✔ Systematic observations have explicit procedures for minimising observer bias, leading to reliable findings

✔ A participant observer is able to gather many contextual details that help to produce a holistic understanding of the site

DISADVANTAGES

✗ Observed behaviours can be open to interpretation. The interpretive framework needs to be made explicit, whether structured or participant observation is used

✗ Systematic observations may not pick up important contextual factors that explain the observed behaviour

✗ Participant observers may gather important contextual data, but what they see and how they interpret that is greatly influenced by the researchers' personal characteristics

✗ The ideal is to observe things 'as they are in their natural state'. However, the very act of situating an observer in the site may change the behaviour of those being observed

✗ Ethics of covert observation must be addressed, in particular the ethical requirement for informed consent

References

Croll P 1986 Systematic classroom observation. Falmer, London

Lofland J, Lofland L 1995 Analysing social settings: a guide to qualitative observation and analysis. Wadsworth, Belmont, CA

Spradley J 1980 Participant observation. Rinehart & Winston, New York

Analysis and presentation

Introduction to analysis

15

The actual approach to analysis will be determined by the research question and the strategy adopted. Surveys require a different approach to ethnography, and case studies will not be analysed in the same way as an experiment. Each tradition has 'rules' that guide the analytic process and ultimately these are used to judge the soundness of the research. Now this is important, as these rules are related to different sets of assumptions about the world and how research should be conducted. This means that the rules determining the soundness of research within one tradition may not hold up when viewed from the perspective of another tradition. For example, within experimental research great emphasis is placed upon objectivity and the researcher remaining detached and not biasing the findings whereas in many kinds of qualitative research the reflexivity of the researcher – i.e. the researcher's own explicit subjectivity – is an important part of establishing the validity of the work.

Analyses of words and numbers are not mutually exclusive and it is not unusual for a case study to include numerical calculations or for surveys based on closed answer questions that will be quantitatively analysed also to include open-ended questions that require some form of qualitative analysis. What is important is that the analytic strategy accords with the overall aims and conceptual framework of the research.

It is at the design stage that your approach to analysis should be clarified. Failing to consider adequately how you intend to analyse your data may lead to a mass of useless, unanalysable words or numbers. You should take guidance at the earliest possible stage so that data can be collected in the most appropriate form. For quantitative data it is important to know which statistical tests you intend to perform on your data. The actual running of the tests is reasonably straightforward within computer software packages, but knowing which tests to apply and the kinds of data that will need to be collected is crucial. Whenever possible, discuss your plans with someone who has expertise in statistics before consolidating your plans for data collection.

There are a variety of approaches to the analysis of qualitative data, from grounded theory to narrative analysis. The kinds of data to be collected, as well as how they are treated, depends on the framework of analysis, which is in turn defined by the questions guiding the research. For example, if you are trying to develop a theory for understanding how individuals make healthcare choices, then a grounded theory approach may be appropriate. If, on the other

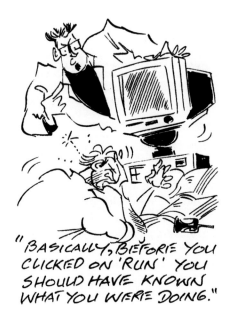

"BASICALLY, BEFORE YOU CLICKED ON 'RUN' YOU SHOULD HAVE KNOWN WHAT YOU WERE DOING."

hand, you want to create an account of one person's experience of an illness and use of healthcare interventions, then a narrative analysis may be a better choice. There are various software packages that can be used to assist in the analysis of qualitative data, however, they do not do the analysis for you in the sense that a statistics package would perform the statistical tests on your quantitative data. The software helps to organise and present the data, with some packages offering more advanced features that will scrutinise the data in relation to specific questions that you pose. There will be a learning curve in getting to know how to use the software, particularly the more sophisticated packages. For small projects, say with data from 20 interviews, the time spent on learning how to use the software may not be a sufficient trade-off for ease of organisation, unless the researcher intends to carry out further projects.

Analysing qualitative data

16

INTRODUCTION

There are a variety of approaches when it comes to analysing qualitative data. Disciplines such as anthropology, sociology and linguistics, to name a few, have developed their own distinctive techniques for working with text, visual and other non-numerical data. These distinctions are mostly related to the different orientation and perspectives within each discipline.

The decision on which methodological stance to take is linked to the framing of the research question. The framework provides a basis for the specific questions you ask, what sort of data you will need to collect, and how you will bring those data together within the analysis. Describing your conceptual framework helps make explicit the assumptions and underlying principles shaping the study. It allows you to lay out the 'givens' and terms of reference, whether they be specific theories you have adopted to view the phenomena, such as psychodynamics, or named methods such as phenomenology, narrative analysis or hermeneutics (see Ch. 2, General design issues).

You may find yourself trying to locate your study within one of the named traditions, such as grounded theory (Glaser & Strauss 1967) or phenomenology (Moustakas 1994). If the research question, conceptual framework and specific methods are all congruent this is fine, but sometimes the research question and the framework for understanding the phenomena demand a more flexible approach to these formal theoretical traditions.

The pressing concern for most small-scale researchers is to devise a method for answering their specific research questions, while the distinctions between the different methodological perspectives tends to be of greater interest to academics and specialists. It is easy to be drawn into perspectives that are so well articulated within the named traditions, but you need to take care this is not at the expense of defining the unique perspective that helped you formulate your research question. What is important is to develop a coherence between your research question, the conceptual framework and the methods you use. In practice you may simply draw on aspects of the named traditions, in service of answering the questions that are important to you as a practitioner. You must have clearly articulated the theories that underpin your own approach to analysis.

The following section will describe a range of tactics that can be used to analyse qualitative data. You would be unlikely to call on all of them in any one study and some only make sense when applied to specific questions; for instance, identifying key events might be more important in developing a narrative account or case study, but if the aim of the study is to map a range of opinions on a particular topic then identifying themes and patterns as well as comparing and contrasting are likely to be more useful tactics. There is not one correct way to analyse qualitative data, but some features such as coding and categorisation are generally applicable.

If the data generated have been in the form of interviews, then these will need to be transcribed. See the section on transcribing in Chapter 12, Interviews, for a discussion of the issues here.

USING COMPUTER SOFTWARE

You will need to decide at a fairly early stage whether or not you intend to use computer software specifically designed for analysing qualitative data. There is a range of programs available, such as Ethnograph (for PC), HyperQual (for Mac and PC), and QRSNUDIST (PC). Each of the programs has somewhat different features and internal logic, but in the end they help to organise, analyse and present data. The question usually hinges on whether the advantages the software can offer in terms of organising, searching, linking and presenting the data are worth the time and effort required in learning how to use the technology competently. For a small-scale researcher who expects to have 20 hours of transcribed interview data the answer is probably not, unless you are very comfortable and efficient at working with new software. Some of the programs are quite sophisticated and allow hyperlinks to text/images and video as well as having complex search and retrieval functions, and for larger projects it probably makes sense to invest the time, effort and money required. But make no mistake, the programs are unable to do the essential work of the analyst. Analysis requires an understanding of context and implied meanings as well as an ability to make intuitive leaps. What the programs can do is help with the mechanical tasks of organising and arranging data.

Some researchers feel much more comfortable working with cards or cut-out passages, quotes and images laid out on the floor or a table, arguing that being able to work with the data spatially helps them in the analytical process. Other researchers, more comfortable working with technology, value highly the search and link functions of the computer software.

BREAKING THE DATA DOWN INTO UNITS

Once you have the data in front of you in the form of transcribed interviews, questionnaires, fieldnotes, images or other artefacts, you will need to organise this for the purposes of analysis. Box 16.1 summarises the main steps involved in this process. The first step is called coding, when the data are broken down into units. These units may be words, phrases or whole passages (or images). It may not be clear what criteria you should use for coding, but in the earliest stages it does not matter too much as the process is subject to constant revision. Background knowledge, professional experience, impressions and hunches can help you break the data down into units. The aim of the research will also guide you; for example, if you are developing a narrative account you will be identifying units of meaning in relation to a life story. If, on the other hand, the aim is to explain the difficulties that can occur in patient–practitioner relationships, then the units might relate to social conventions and practices, roles, events, thoughts, opinions and strategies. The important point is that each unit of data should be the smallest piece of information that can stand by itself without losing the thread of meaning it had in the context in which it appeared.

Box 16.1 Basic steps in analysing qualitative data

- Coding the data by breaking it down into units of meaning
- Conceptually categorising the content of each unit
- Developing or tracing themes or patterns
- Reconstructing as narrative or more general theory
- Justifying the methods and conclusions – validity claims in terms of the research aims and conceptual framework; accounting for bias, challenging the interpretations – triangulation, negative instances, rival explanations, member checking

---

IDENTIFYING CATEGORIES

As you examine the data you will probably recognise that many of the units of data are similar or relate to each other in some way, i.e. they fall into clusters or categories. The data may be from an individual interview or from a wider data set. These clusters or categories should be grouped together — physically on cards, cut-out photocopies or within a computer program. This process of organising the data into categories can start as soon as the data come in. The categories at this stage are tentative and provisional and based on your earliest impressions of what the data contain. The research question and the conceptual framework will have a pervasive influence on what you see in the data, and if you have conducted a series of semi-structured interviews you will probably find many of the responses fall into categories related to the specific areas covered. It is important to stay open to the possibility that the data may not fall neatly into predictable categories and using a combination of your background knowledge, intuitive leaps and a playful approach to the data you may find other potential categories emerging. This is not the stage to be overly rigid. As the process goes on there will be opportunities to refine, consolidate or eliminate your tentative formulations.

As you start to gather units of data that seem to be referring to the same or similar things, you can begin to define what that particular category is about. Try writing a propositional statement about the category. This category definition in a sense sets the inclusion and exclusion criteria that will allow you to judge whether a particular piece of data belongs in this category or another one. This is where you begin to theorise about the data. When you group items together by their common features you are making a theoretical abstraction.

You may well find that you need to adjust, amend and refine the category definition in light of new data coming in. Some categories may need to merge under a new definition and others may be further divided into sub-categories. The data within the categories should be internally consistent, while the categories themselves should be clearly distinct and differentiated from each other.

THEMES AND PATTERNS

A step further in theoretical development is to look for the relationships between the categories and any patterns that link the categories together. Some of the linkages come from explicit statements in the data. The people you are studying will have their own sense-making processes, whether it be identifying causes and effects or other kinds of relationships. These may be helpful as a starting point; however, the analyst will not simply accept these interpretations but will look further into the data for patterns that may not be obvious. Once again your previous experience, the conceptual framework and the specific research question help you to 'see' patterns in the data. You should be clear about whether you are trying to *describe, explain, compare, trace* or *predict* something about your topic. In tracing out themes and patterns you will also look for the plausibility of the linkages. Ask yourself whether these patterns make sense and if they can be verified in any way.

If you are working with hard copy you can lay out the piles of data in some sort of spatial relationship on a table or the floor and make some theoretical statements about the linkages between the categories. A similar process can take place on screen within the software programs (see section on narrative analysis, p. 174 below, for a different take on this process).

There are certain questions you can ask about the relationships between the data that can help develop your understanding. You should examine the data for the conditions under which the properties of the category are pronounced or minimised, the consequences of these variations and how such variations in the properties of one category impact upon the properties of other categories. You are trying to unpack the relationships between the categories by noting under what conditions they vary. For instance, in interviews with asthma patients where you are interested in how they manage their condition you may have a category relating to 'seeking professional advice'. A range of factors may influence when advice is sought and when and how it is acted upon. By going back to the data again and again you ensure that the theoretical links made are not pie in the sky. You may find that the data do not have all the answers to your questions, but if the analysis starts as soon as the data come in, then future data collection cycles can be oriented towards answering the questions that emerge through the analysis. This working back and forth between the data and the analysis ensures that theoretical development is grounded in the real world (Glaser & Strauss 1967).

To further your understanding of what the data may contain there are a range of tactics that you can call upon. Miles and Hubberman (1994) provide a useful discussion on the following: noting patterns and themes, seeing plausibility, clustering, making metaphors, counting, making comparisons and contrasts, partitioning variables, subsuming particulars into the general, factoring, noting relationships between variables, building a logical chain of evidence, making conceptual/theoretical coherence. It is worth examining some of these tactics in more detail.

METAPHORS

Using metaphors is a useful way of making conceptual links within the data. A metaphor draws out the similarities while ignoring the differences between the two things being compared. To describe a friend as a rock calls forth the solidity and enduring qualities of the friendship, whilst ignoring all the obvious differences such as sentience, communicability, etc. Metaphors can help us to understand and make theoretical links within our data in the same way that the people we study use them to make sense of their own experience. A metaphor highlights particular aspects of the phenomenon being described and at the same time opens the possibility to see aspects that may not have been obvious without the metaphorical association. In that way they can help identify new linkages within the data. It is worth being conscious of the metaphors that appear within the data as well as the metaphors that you use yourself. These can be mined (to use a metaphor) for associations and deeper meanings. Lakoff and Johnson (1980) provide a useful discussion about the way ordinary reasoning is based on metaphorical association. While metaphors can help in making links and developing theory, we should be cautious about pushing the metaphors too far or accepting them uncritically. Better to think of them as a springboard for conceptual development that will then need to be carefully examined to tease out where the associations start and finish.

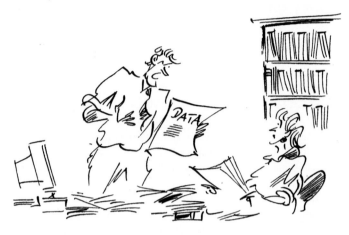

" IT NEEDS MORE THAN A MASSAGE — TRY A CHIROPRACTOR. "

COUNTING

Although the term qualitative is by definition non-numerical, counting can be an important part of making qualitative judgements. Miles and Hubberman (1994) describe three good reasons to examine the frequency of occurrences in the data. The first is to assess rapidly what the data contain. The second is to verify a hunch or hypothesis and the third is to protect against biases that might obscure or amplify particular aspects of the data. Simple frequency counts rather than complex calculations or statistics will usually suffice. To know that 16 out of 20 respondents gave an affirmative response to a particular question is a more specific way of expressing a general tendency.

BUILDING EXPLANATIONS

From identifying the linkages between individual categories you will need to go on and explain how these linkages hang together. You are looking for an explanation or story that makes sense of the discrete categories and links them together in a meaningful way. Your explanation or theory will need to have a clearly discernible logic; however, by itself a compelling logic is insufficient. You must carefully verify each link in the logic chain by going

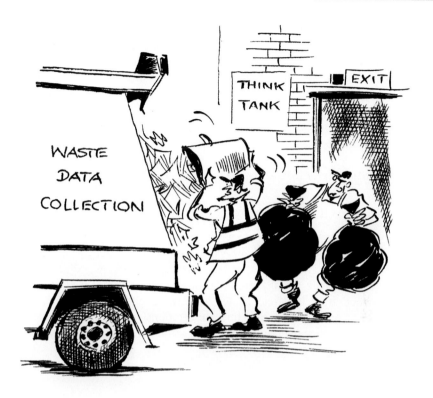

back to the data for confirmation. You should ask not only whether there is some evidence to support the links in your explanation but whether there is evidence that contradicts or falls outside your explanatory logic or whether there are gaps in the data that make your links purely speculative. If the analysis is taking place concurrently with data collection, then future rounds of data collection can be directed towards filling the data gaps or challenging the interpretations you have made by looking for contradictory evidence.

If there is an inadequate fit between the data and your explanations you should modify and refine your explanation to accommodate the actual data that have been gathered. Lincoln and Guba (1985) refer to this as negative case analysis, where instances or 'cases' that do not fit the emerging theory lead to a revision of the theory until all the 'cases' are accounted for. There is a dance that takes place between data and theory, a dynamic working back and forth between the meaning you see in the data and what evidence you have to support that view. You can explore whether alterative explanations provide a more convincing fit to the data, but you should bear in mind the purpose you want that theory to serve. There is always more that one way of interpreting data, what is important is that the theory you work with helps you address the intellectual or practical puzzle driving your research.

The analysis is built by moving back and forth from the interrelationships between categories to broader constructs and theories that explain the hows and whys of the phenomena you are studying. The concepts and theories may come specifically from your professional field or from other disciplines. The movement is from specific and local constructs that explain particular interrelationships to more encompassing theories.

Through the process of analysis the researcher will draw on theory to: recognise the common features of data as they are separated into categories, make links between the data categories, recognise patterns and themes, and explain the significance of these patterns.

MAPS AND CHARTS

It can be helpful to create visual representations of your explanation, whether in the form of diagrams, flow charts, matrices, maps or webs of relationships. The process of abstracting or reducing your analysis to relatively simple visual representations can be a useful way of discerning the wood from the trees. Flow charts are a concise way of representing processes and matrices can show the relationships between variables. Maps can be used to show relationships and influences and can help you identify where your data and evidence are strongest and where they might be lacking.

NARRATIVE ANALYSIS

In contrast to themes and patterns identified from a series of interviews, a narrative analysis will keep data relating to an individual embedded in the specific and particular context of that person's life story. The analyst will string together the narrative components of the transcript as well as identifying other forms of data within a transcript. As well as having a temporal sequence, narrative forms are oriented by structures such as plot, key characters (heroes, villains etc.), defining events and influential factors. The analysis goes beyond a factual reconstruction of events to explore the meanings and social processes that define and shape the narrative. Some of the tactics described above (making metaphors, noting relationships between variables, building a convincing chain of logic) can help move the narrative beyond the descriptive level (Mishler 1991). The analyst is not simply searching for the 'true story', as the precise content as well as the presentation of every narrative is determined by the context of its telling. Rather than viewing the narrative as a true representation of events, the analyst uses the narrative as a window to understand the individual and the social forces that shape the telling of the story (Mattingly 1991).

REFLEXIVITY

Throughout the analytic process the researcher will be reflecting on the significance of the data. It is important to maintain a record of these

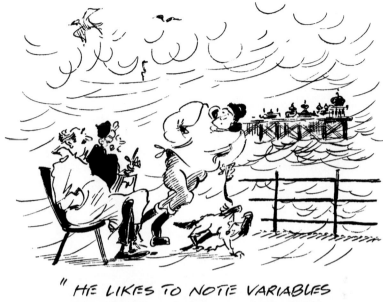

" HE LIKES TO NOTE VARIABLES
AND BUILD A CONVINCING CHAIN
OF LOGIC ~ BUT I'M JUST HAPPY
WATCHING THE TIDE COMING IN. "

reflections as the analytic process is an interplay between the data themselves and the researcher's own subjectivity. These reflections or memos may be logged in a diary and consist of questions, insights and developing lines of thinking.

The researcher should also refer to memos recorded in the design and data collection phases of the research. These memos become data that feed into the analytic process (see section on reflexivity, p. 72 in Ch. 7, Ethnography).

JUSTIFYING YOUR METHODS AND CONCLUSIONS

There is a range of criteria for judging the soundness of qualitative research. Some of these criteria are shared with quantitative research and others are more specific to qualitative research. In essence, the judgements are about the validity or truth value of the research. It is a reasonable expectation that research is honest, credible and trustworthy, but the basis for making these judgements is not so simple and self-evident.

Objectivity

The 'rules' generally applied to quantitative research are rooted in a 'realist' assumption that the world can be studied objectively. This is linked to the assumption that knowledge should have a high degree of correspondence with a single objective reality. From this perspective knowledge should mirror that objective reality — free from the distortions of poor instrumentation and human bias. A contrasting perspective held by qualitative researchers is that knowledge is always the product of human and social forces. These forces will shape how research questions are formulated as well as the selective perception process that turns the mass of incoming sense data into meaningful chunks and orders them. This is a more 'relativist' position, that acknowledges the way a researcher's previous experience, background knowledge, preferences and prejudices will have an influential effect on what the researcher 'sees' and how this is interpreted. This is not to suggest that qualitative research by definition lacks rigour, but that the rules for evaluating the research have to take account of the way these human and social forces impact on the work.

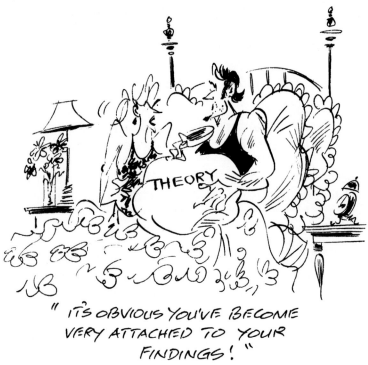

" IT'S OBVIOUS YOU'VE BECOME
VERY ATTACHED TO YOUR
FINDINGS ! "

Validity

Validity is about the truth value of the research. From a qualitative research perspective this means establishing defensible knowledge claims rather than a search for an absolute singular truth.

AIM

Validity must be seen in relation to the aims of the research. If the aim is to develop an explanation of a social phenomenon, then a primary validity question will be whether the logic of the interpretation is sound and whether the conceptual framework is appropriate to answer such a question and analyse the incoming data. If the aim is to find new ways of thinking about or acting in relation to a specific problem, then the conceptual framework and interpretation must be appropriate for this task. This is pragmatic validity — how effective is the analysis in providing a guide for action? This kind of validity is established in the field of action and is a central validity criterion within traditions such as action research.

FROM DESIGN TO REPORTING

Validity is not established by following a set of defined quality control procedures. It is a continual process of checking, questioning and theoretically interpreting through every phase of the research from design to reporting. Rather than attempting to show your analysis is the only possible one, your aim should be to demonstrate convincingly that, given the position you have adopted, and the evidence you present, a reader can see your justification for the analysis. You will need to demonstrate convincingly how your analysis evolved. You should not take as self-evident that your particular interpretation is justified; rather, your reporting should provide a systematic charting of how your understanding developed, including how you arrived at the analytic choices you made. This means that the context for your decisions should be explained. This is sometimes referred to as 'thick description' (Geertz 1973), where sufficient detail of the process and context of the analysis allows readers to make their own inferences as well as judge whether those made by the researcher are sound. Thick description also allows the reader to judge how far the findings might be transferable to other settings.

There are no hard and fast methodological rules that guarantee validity. Validity is based on a continual process of checking, questioning and theoretically interpreting through every phase of the research, from design to reporting.

Specific techniques to check validity

There are some specific techniques used within qualitative research to support the validity of the interpretation.

TRIANGULATION

This term refers to the use of multiple data sources, methods of data collection and investigators, in order to corroborate, complement or challenge findings. Each data source, method or investigator can bring a somewhat different perspective to the analysis. Two researchers can check how reliably they independently assign data to specific categories. This inter-rater reliability can be checked using a percentage agreement statistic.

Drawing on multiple data sources about an event can potentially provide stronger evidence than a single source. In a similar way, using multiple methods such as questionnaires as well as in-depth interviews or documentary sources can provide a richer account, and when the findings are corroborated the validity is enhanced. But this should not be accepted naively. A finding that is not corroborated is not by definition false. Nor is it possible to say that when a finding is corroborated it is always true. There can be many reasons for a divergence. Individuals providing data are likely to 'see' events differently through their own preferences and prejudices. Using different methods may lead to contrasting data about the same topic. What an individual might feel able to say within the (perhaps collusive) pressure of a focus group may be quite different from what that person would say in a sensitively conducted one-on-one interview. Using multiple investigators is no guarantee of validity, although it can be a powerful way of challenging interpretations and providing contrasting views.

Triangulation, like other validation strategies, is best thought of as a reflexive device rather than a definitive test. It cannot prove that your data are truthful. The idea of there being one single truth that all the lines of inquiry converge upon (as the two-dimensional geometrical metaphor of triangulation suggests) has little credibility when viewed within the complex human world. Triangulation can encourage you to reflect upon and explore the tensions that exist within your data, and ultimately produce more credible analyses.

MEMBER CHECKS

Another important tool for validating your findings is to check them out with the people on the ground. Lincoln and Guba (1985) suggest that the data, analytic categories, interpretations and conclusions are tested with members of the stakeholding groups from which the data were originally collected. This can take place both informally and/or formally. If the members consider that your reconstructions of their experiences or events are adequate, then this supports the validity of your findings.

Member checking can be part of a continuous process, from verbally summarising the key points of an interview and checking whether this is what the respondent meant, to having respondents check transcripts for accuracy and whether these adequately represent their experiences. What may happen at this point is that specific details may be clarified or even altered. A further step is to provide a tentative report of the analysis and conclusions for respondents' feedback on whether the researcher's construction is fair enough. Their responses can feed back into the analytic process.

While member checking can be a valuable exercise, it cannot be relied upon as the final judge of validity. There could be covert (or open) reasons why members might want their experience, event or organisation presented in a particular way. The researcher needs to be aware of possible political motivations that could sway how members might respond to a report. It is up to you as the researcher to weigh the criticisms made and decide, in light of all the evidence, to present your findings as accurately and fairly as you are able.

Box 16.2   Checking for bias
● Negative instances ● Challenging the interpretations ● Checking the interpretation with those on the ground – member checks ● Adopting devil's advocate position ● Ruling out rival explanations

Challenging your interpretations should be an integral part of the analytic process, not only at the stage of member checking (see Box 16.2). You should examine the data carefully for alternative explanations and cases or instances that do not fit your theory (see section on building explanations, above). It is easy to become attached to one's own theorising and overlook any counter evidence or other possible formulations.

Part of justifying your conclusions is demonstrating how you looked for and dealt with evidence that did not neatly fit your interpretation. You can adopt a devil's advocate position in relation to your theory, or have a colleague do this for you. It can be very helpful to have regular peer debriefing with others not involved in the research in order to reveal your blind spots.

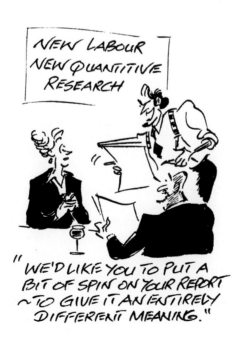

"WE'D LIKE YOU TO PUT A BIT OF SPIN ON YOUR REPORT ~ TO GIVE IT AN ENTIRELY DIFFERENT MEANING."

References

Geertz C 1973 The interpretation of culture: selected essays. Basic Books, New York

Glaser B, Strauss A 1967 The discovery of grounded theory. Aldine, Chicago

Lakoff G, Johnson M 1980 The metaphors we live by. University of Chicago Press, Chicago

Lincoln Y, Guba E 1985 Naturalistic inquiry. Sage, Thousand Oak

Mattingly C 1991 The narrative nature of clinical reasoning. American Journal of Occupational Therapy 45(11): 998–1005

Miles M, Hubberman A 1994 Qualitative data analysis: an expanded source book. Sage, Thousand Oak

Mishler E 1991 Research interviewing: context and narrative. Harvard University Press, Cambridge MA

Moustakas C 1994 Phenomenological research methods. Sage, Thousand Oak

Analysing quantitative data

17

INTRODUCTION

There are many good reasons for using quantitative data, such as ease of manipulation and being able to work with larger data sets without much increase in effort. For some people there is also the mystique of numbers and the belief that good science depends on quantification. While this last point is certainly debatable, it is true that science has developed very sophisticated methods for analysing numerical data and that a great deal of important scientific work has utilised this approach. In this chapter we will introduce some of the basic concepts for understanding and working with numbers. Even if you don't intend to use any statistics within your own study, getting a handle on the basic concepts can help when it comes to critically evaluating published studies.

SIMPLE STATISTICS

Fundamentally, statistics are a set of tools for describing, organising and interpreting numerical data. The basics are suprisingly simple, even for those with numerophobia.

Everyone has grown up learning how to apply some level of statistical understanding.

When we use words like 'I usually have porridge for breakfast' or 'the telephone normally rings whenever I get in the bath' we are making use of

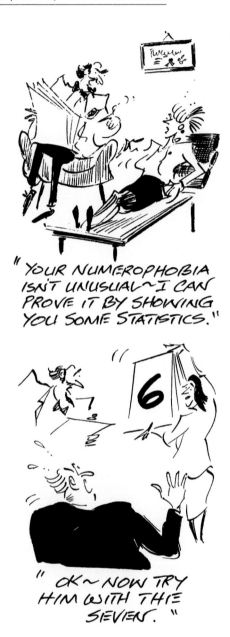

concepts at the heart of statistics. We might even formalise this by saying that there is a 50/50 chance that a bus will come to the stop as soon as I decide to walk on. When we say that we will probably see our friends at the weekend we are making a prediction which statistics can be used to quantify. Statistics takes the meaning of these everyday words and applies mathematical treatment to bring precision to their use. This does not mean that you need to have more than a very basic understanding of mathematics to make use of statistics. Fortunately, there are plenty of computer software packages that can do this part of it for you.

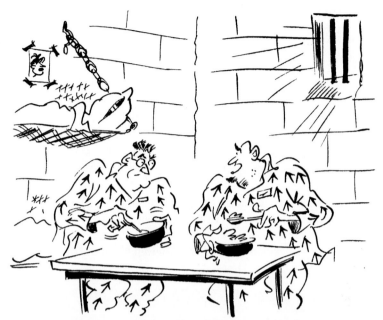

" THE PAST 10 YEARS HAVE TAUGHT ME
THAT I HAVE MORE THAN A 50% CHANCE
OF HAVING PORRIDGE FOR BREAKFAST. "

You may hear a statistic quoted like 13 in 100 school children have been diagnosed with asthma. This does not mean that if we were to count children by the hundred at your local schools, then 13 and only 13 children out of every 100 counted would have asthma. Nor does it tell us which of the 100 children have the disease. It only tells us of the likelihood of this occurring across a population. We grow up thinking in terms of probabilities — the likelihood of rain when we go out, of safety walking at night. We often do what we can to reduce the likelihood of these occurrences — carrying an umbrella, taking a taxi or walking with a friend at night.

CLARIFYING WHAT YOU NEED BEFORE YOU GATHER THE DATA

The inexperienced researcher may set out to gather as much data as possible with the assumption that all the numbers can be crunched later; however, more data do not make better research, and simplicity is a virtue. Especially with experimental work, it is vital to know in advance what forms of data analysis will be performed. Whenever it is feasible, consider consulting a statistician to get advice on the relationship between sample size and the expected difference in effect between the intervention and non-intervention groups. It is very unfortunate when researchers decide to consult a statistician at the analysis stage, when it is too late to rectify any design faults.

WHAT KINDS OF DATA?

Before we go any further it is important to clarify that there are different types of quantitative data. These differences, based on ordering and ranking, are important and will determine which statistical tests you can meaningfully apply and the conclusions you will be able to draw.

Nominal data

This is the most basic form of quantitative data and is generated when you count and categorise things. For example:

- sex — female, male
- religion — buddhist, christian, jew, hindu
- occupation — butcher, baker, candlestick maker.

There is no underlying order or relationship between the categories, which are based simply on the names.

Ordinal data

Ordinal data are generated by counting the frequency of the occurrences but unlike nominal data, each category is, as the name suggests, ordered and ranked in a scale. An example is a pain scale ranging from: no pain — mild pain — moderate pain — severe pain — extreme pain.

Each of the above categories can be laid out in relation to each other, but this form of data provides no quantification of how great the difference is between the categories, or whether there is a greater difference between, say, extreme and severe pain or mild and no pain.

Interval data

Interval data are ranked like ordinal data, but the differences between the categories are quantifiable; for example, the hours of the day, in which the intervals are all the same. These measurable differences allow more refined statistical manipulation.

Ratio data

Ratio data are like interval data in having categories that are proportionate, but these proportions are in relation to an absolute point. For example, weight and height have absolute zero points. It makes no sense to refer to less than 0 height.

Continuous data

There are some kinds of interval and ratio data where differences are on a continuum, such as time, height or weight. For practical purposes these are grouped to the nearest unit. Although in principle it is possible to measure the differences down to the millisecond, millimetre or milligram, this kind of precision may not be necessary or available, and dealing with vast categories of data creates unnecessary complications in analysis. It may be sufficient to know or round up the height to the nearest centimetre, or the time taken to complete a task to the nearest second or minute, depending on the nature of the study. The researcher who sets the boundaries of the categories will need to be very clear in defining where the boundaries and midpoints of the categories are, as these are used in statistically manipulating continuous data.

ORGANISING THE DATA

Coding

For some variables such as age or IQ (continuous variables) it is possible simply to enter the number measured. If the data we are collecting do not naturally occur in numbers (nominal and ordinal data), we must assign codes. The coding process gives a numerical value to words, observations or whatever units constitute the data. Nominal data such as gender or religion are given an arbitrary numerical value such as 0 or 1 to aid in the manipulation of the data. With ordinal data a numerical scheme is created, such as 0-1-2-3-4-5 in the pain scale referred to earlier, with 0 signifying no pain and 5 signifying extreme pain. With nominal data the numbers do not indicate how great the difference is between the possible categories. For interval and ratio data, the code numbers represent precise and measurable differences between each category. From continuous data the researcher is able to define the categories, such as ages 10-19, 20-29, 30-39, 40-49 and above, for ease of analysis. Again for ease in analysis, each of these categories can be assigned a number, such as category 1 for ages 10-19, category 2 for 20-29, etc.

It is important when developing a coding frame that there is no overlap between each of the codes — this means a response should fit only one category and no other. The range of codes should also be comprehensive, to cover the range of possible responses. This raises the question whether the coding frame should be developed at the design stage or post-data collection. Developing a coding frame in the design stage allows the individual questions in a questionnaire to be pre-coded, making the analysis simpler. If the study is exploratory, the full range of responses may not be known, so the coding frame will have to be developed in light of the incoming data. While this flexibility allows the development of new categories, the disadvantage is that post-collection coding is quite time-consuming. A compromise is having an 'other — please specify' box, where respondents to a questionnaire can provide answers that do not fit the pre-coded categories. However, if more responses fall in the 'other' category than in the pre-coded responses, this indicates an insufficient number of categories. On the other hand, having too many categories that have infrequent responses only complicates the analysis, and a balance needs to be struck here (see sections on coding in Ch. 8, Experiments and quasi-experiments, and Ch. 13, Questionnaires).

Once coded, the data are ready for analysis. Basic counting of frequencies and amounts is a key step, and this requires nothing more complex mathematically than addition. Important research findings may depend on this level of analysis alone, but frequently researchers will want to subject their data to somewhat more demanding statistical analysis. Software packages such as Statistical Package for Social Scientists (SPSS) provide a range of options for analysing coded data, without obliging the researcher to understand how to perform the complex mathematics behind the statistics. However, it is important that you understand which tests are appropriate for the data you have collected (and for answering your research question). This requires a basic understanding of how statistics are applied. Statistics may be used to provide detailed descriptions of the data (descriptive statistics), as well as to allow us to draw conclusions about the population of interest from the study of a sample (inferential statistics).

PRESENTING THE DATA

There are various statistical software packages such as SPSS that allow the user to code and recode the data for statistical analysis. There is also software that assists the user in presenting the data in the form of tables and graphs. Salkind (2000) provides a brief overview of key features. These packages offer a wide choice for visual presentation, but a key principle is to keep the table or graph simple. Of course there is considerable effort required in learning how to use the software competently. Salkind (2000) provides a useful basic introduction to using SPSS. You should avoid the temptation to fit more and more information into your table or graph, and include only the essentials for conveying the point you wish to get across. Less is often more when it comes to presenting tables or graphs.

Descriptive statistics

AVERAGES

One of the main functions of statistics is to describe sets of numbers concisely, yet accurately. This is achieved by summarising data in terms of averages and examining the degree of variation around that average (standard deviation). The average is a summary of a larger set of numbers. But there is more than one kind of average. These different measures can produce very different results. They are all known as measures of central tendency.

The mean (the arithmetical average)

If you read a report that says that the average weight of men in their 20s in the UK has increased from 70 kg in 1900 to 80 kg in 2000, simplistically you

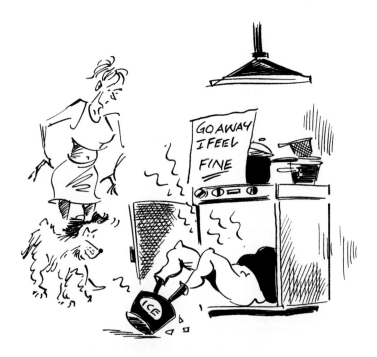

might assume that the weight of each and every person had proportionately increased. But clearly weight gains are not evenly distributed.

The mean is inappropriate to use with nominal data, as the concept of 'average' doesn't apply to discrete categories. It is also worth bearing in mind that the mean can be pulled towards extreme scores. That is, if the times taken to run a mile by a group of 20 boys were all less than 7 minutes, except for one who took 20 minutes, this would seriously skew the mean average of the group towards a longer time than all but one of the boys ran.

The mode

In the above example it might be more appropriate to refer to the mode. The *mode* is the most commonly occurring score in the data set. If, for instance, 12 of the boys ran the mile in 6 minutes and seven boys ran it in 5 minutes, then the mode would be 6 minutes. It is used in preference to the mean as the measure of central tendency when the data are skewed, as it is less sensitive to the distorting effect of extreme scores.

The median

The *median* divides the distribution into half; half of the scores fall under the median and half above the median. The median is literally the halfway point between a group of numbers. It is sometimes used in preference to the mean, being less sensitive to the distorting effect of extreme scores.

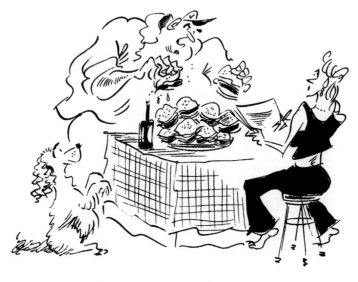

" SORRY, BUT I'M NOT GOING ON A DIET TO FIDDLE YOUR MEAN. "

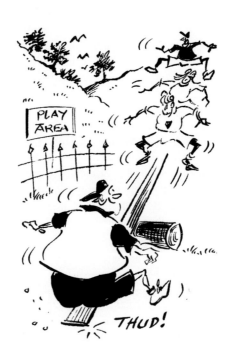

THE SPREAD OF DATA

The average is a measure of central tendency, but it is often useful to know how the data set as a whole is spread out. There are several ways of describing this variance.

The range

The range is the most general measure of variability. It is the difference between the highest and lowest scores. To calculate the range of 10, 14, 15, 16, 17 and 25 you would subtract 10, the lowest score, from 25, the highest score, to come up with a range of 15. Although this statistic has its uses, it is limited by the fact that it is very sensitive to the effect of extreme scores. It is the measures of central tendency that are useful for telling us the point around which most of the scores lie. Measures of spread are useful to show how variable the scores are.

Fractiles

By dividing the range up into fractions around the median, comparisons can be made about the spread of scores. The fractions can vary, but quarters are commonly used. This is achieved by subdividing the range into four evenly distributed parts. Each quartile has exactly one quarter of all the scores, allowing the researcher to identify and work with the middle half of all scores. This is known as the interquartile range (those between 25% and 75%). Deciles divide the range into tenths, which can be useful in making comparisons about the different subgroups, such as the highest and lowest scores (Fig. 17.1).

Standard deviation

The standard deviation describes the average spread of data around the mean. Rather than relying on highest and lowest scores alone, all the scores together are used to calculate the spread around the mean. In simple terms it is the

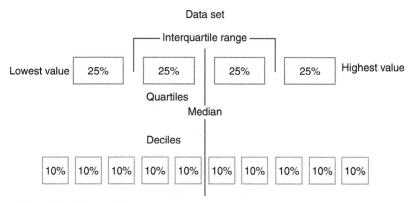

Figure 17.1 Quartiles and deciles.

average distance from the mean. The larger the standard deviation, the greater the spread of the total scores. Like the mean, the standard deviation can be skewed by extreme scores. All in all though, the standard deviation is an extremely useful calculation and is often used as part of more complex statistical calculations. The practical part of calculating the standard deviation is performed very simply within statistical software packages, and the project researcher need not worry too much about how the calculation is done manually but should be very clear about when it should be used. It is suitable for interval and ratio data, but not for nominal or ordinal data as it is based on a calculation of the mean. There is, of course, no mean of nominal or ordinal data.

Inferential statistics

As well as summarising and describing data, statistics can be used to examine the data for links and associations. Inferential statistics help to establish whether associations we 'see', expect or predict will be in the data are actually there. Using the data we collect from our sample, it is possible to make inferences about the study population. Using probability theory, inferential statistics help us make judgements about how confident we can be that what we have found in our data set can be applied to the whole study population (see Ch. 11, Sampling).

> *Statistical inference is the use of probability theory to make inferences about a population from sample data.*

CONFIDENCE INTERVALS

When you calculate descriptive statistics it is normally based on a sample rather than the whole population, and is therefore prone to a degree of error (see Ch. 11, Sampling). The confidence interval is the interval around the estimated mean which we can be confident contains the true population mean. This calculation, using the size, mean and standard deviation of the sample, is based on the assumption of normal distribution (see p. 191 below on distribution of data), i.e. that the sample was selected randomly and that each score is independent of each other.

SIGNIFICANCE LEVEL

Rather than giving absolute and unequivocal answers, inferential statistics tell us how probable it is that the findings were due to random or chance factors. If the chances were only 50/50, then you would not give much credibility to the findings. One in 100 would be far more convincing. There is a generally accepted convention in science that if the chances of the findings being due to random factors are less than five in 100 (5%, one in 20 or, in the language of statistics, $p < 0.05$), then they should be taken seriously. Accepting a set of results as significant could be what is known as a type I error when in fact the particular results were due to random variation. However, at a significance level of 0.05 the likelihood of this occurring is only 5%. A type II error would be to accept incorrectly that the results were due to chance factors rather than a real effect.

Statisticians may mean something different from the rest of us when they use familiar language. In normal English, 'significant' means important, while in statistics 'significant' means probably true (not due to chance). A research finding may be true without being important. When statisticians say a result is 'highly significant' they mean it is very probably true. They do not (necessarily) mean it is highly important.

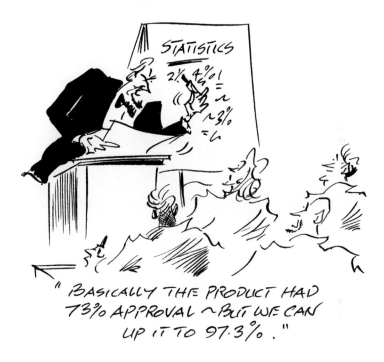

" BASICALLY THE PRODUCT HAD 73% APPROVAL ~BUT WE CAN UP IT TO 97.3% . "

There are a number of tests that you can use on your data to check for significance, such as the chi square test, the t-test and the Mann–Whitney U test. Which tests you should use will depend on the type of data (nominal, ordinal, interval and ratio) as well as on how the scores of the data are spread.

DISTRIBUTION OF DATA

There are some characteristic ways that data tend to be distributed. Quite often the greatest concentration of scores will be in the middle rather than at the extremes. This is not to suggest that this is always the case, but a normal distribution occurs when the mean, median and mode are roughly equal. The best way of examining the distribution of scores is to plot them on a curve. If the curve is bell-shaped, this indicates a distribution that is described as normal (Figs 17.2a, b). For example, if we were to weigh a sample of British men we would find that there would be hardly any who weighed between 0 and 40 kg,

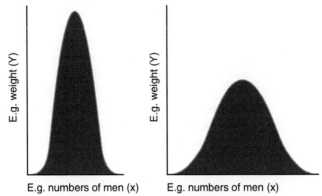

Figure 17.2a   Examples of normal distribution curves.

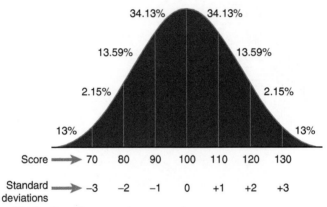

Figure 17.2b   Distribution of cases under a normal curve.

somewhat more between 41 and 70 kg, many more between 71 and 90 kg, somewhat fewer between 91 and 120 kg and very few between 121 and 200 kg.

Certainly not all data sets have this sort of distribution. Sometimes it is skewed to one extreme or the other, or may even have peaks. To determine the shape of the distribution, the distance of each individual score from the mean of all the scores is calculated. If there are more negative distances than positive, then the data are positively skewed, since the mean is being pulled away from the median by a small number of large values. For example, a negative skew has the long tail to the left, indicating a greater concentration of higher scores, and the positive skew is the converse, with the long tail to the right (Fig. 17.3). Some statistical tests, such as the t-test, are only valid with a normal distribution of data, so it is important to check the distribution before you decide on which inferential statistics you use. To examine the distribution of your data the individual scores are measured for their distance from the mean of your total scores.

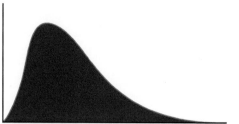

Positive skew has greatest concentration of higher scores to the left

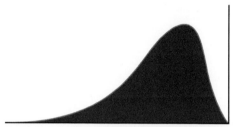

Negative skew has greatest concentration of higher scores to the right

Figure 17.3   Positive and negative skew.

CORRELATION CO-EFFICIENTS

Correlation is the extent to which one thing varies with another. An example of this is the ends of a see-saw: as one end goes up the other end goes down. This is a perfect negative (or inverse) correlation, the degree of upward movement at one end corresponding precisely with the degree of downward movement at the other end.

Expressed in terms of correlation co-efficients, a perfect positive is expressed as 1, no correlation at all is indicated by 0 and a perfect negative is −1. On the scatterplot a perfect positive or negative correlation would appear as a straight line, something very unusual when examining things in the human world. A zero correlation would show as no discernible pattern on the scatterplot (Figs 17.4a,b,c). Interval or ratio data are required for these calculations.

CHI SQUARE

The chi square test assesses the probability of an apparent relationship being due to chance factors alone. This is achieved by placing the data into contingency tables and comparing your data to the values you might expect if there were no relationship between the variables. It is an index of the discrepancy between the recorded and expected scores. The test assumes that if there were no relationship between the variables, then the scores would be evenly distributed throughout the contingency tables (each piece of data from

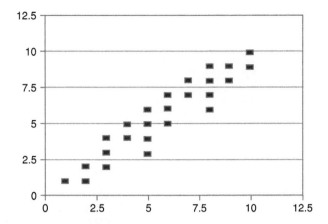

Figure 17.4a   High positive correlation.

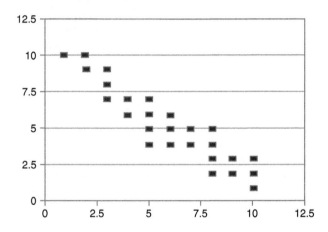

Figure 17.4b   High negative correlation.

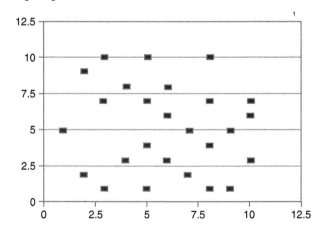

Figure 17.4c   No correlation.

the sample appearing only once in the contingency table). The chi square test can be used on nominal, ordinal, ratio and interval data and does not depend on the data having a normal distribution. Although the chi square test can be used on relatively small data sets, statisticians advise against using it when expected frequencies within the cells of the table are very low, say 5 in a small table. There are other tests, such as Fisher's Exact Test, that can be substituted in such cases.

t-TEST

If you need to compare two sets of data to see whether there is a significant difference between them, you can use the t-test. You may want to compare the scores before and after an intervention. For example, you may want to establish whether a treatment has made any difference to a condition being treated. You would have two sets of data — those taken before the intervention and those taken after. The t-test uses the mean and standard deviation from the two sets of data to come up with a figure that expresses the likelihood that any differences between the two data sets are due to chance alone. This would be expressed as a probability. The convention is that we accept a one in 20 (or $p < 0.05$) chance of making a mistake when we say that an observed effect is real, rather than due to sampling variation. In this way, if p is less than 0.05 we say the result is significant. The great strength of the t-test is that it can be used with small samples and data sets that are not exactly equal in size. The t-test assumes a normal distribution (bell shaped), and a small sample with a skewed distribution could lead to misleading results. It also assumes the same degree of variability between the two populations from which the samples were taken. There are variations on the t-test, depending on whether the data sets are matched. The paired two group t-test is a variation in which it is possible to pair each of the pre- and post-intervention scores. The unpaired two group t-test is used when such pairing is not possible. When presenting the results of t-tests, the t-value and the probability of the result being due to chance (p value), as well as the mean and standard deviation of the two sets of scores, are included. Most statistics packages will offer this choice and generate such tables automatically. The great strength of the t-test is that it can be used with small samples and data sets of unequal size. Table 17.1 gives an example of a t-test table.

There is a wide range of statistical methods that can be used to summarise data as well as to detect relationships between variables, and only the basic ones have been introduced in this chapter. Each statistical test has an appropriate use as well as limitations. It is important that you understand what kinds of tests can be applied to your data, and how they will help you answer your research questions. It is wise to seek advice from someone with statistical expertise at the design stage. The actual calculation of the statistics is handled very simply within statistical software packages; what is most crucial is knowing why the tests are being applied.

Table 17.1 Example of a *t*-test table (Peter Davies, unpublished, with permission)											
Hours of sleep of 10 patients were observed before and after taking "Sleep-ease", a new herbal remedy											
Patient	1	2	3	4	5	6	7	8	9	10	Mean
After	6.1	7.0	8.2	7.6	6.5	8.4	6.9	6.7	7.4	5.8	7.06
Before	5.2	7.9	3.9	4.7	5.3	5.4	4.2	6.1	3.8	6.3	5.28
Difference	0.9	−0.9	4.3	2.9	1.2	3.0	2.7	0.6	3.6	−0.5	1.78

References

Salkind N 2000 Statistics for people who (think they) hate statistics. Sage, Thousand Oak

Further reading

There is a wide variety of resources to further your understanding of statistics.
Huff D 1991 How to lie with statistics. Penguin, London
This is a very accessible primer.
Rowntree D 2000 Statistics without tears. Penguin, Harmondsworth
Salkind N 2000 Statistics for people who (think they) hate statistics. Sage, Thousand Oak
These are useful introductory texts, even for numerophobes.

Websites

HyperStat online tutorials http://www.davidmlane.com/hyperstat/
Selecting statistics http://biochim.human.cornell.edu/selstat/ssstart.htm
There are plenty of websites devoted to statistics, some of these providing basic courses and online software for making calculations.

Writing up

Writing up

18

INTRODUCTION

Writing up your research project is the culmination of many months of intense effort in which you create a formal record of the research endeavour. It is tempting to consider the research complete when you have the data in and it is analysed, but writing up is much more than rote recording of what has taken place and what was found. It is in writing up that you give expression to your learning and where you document for others how that learning took place and the significance of what was found. The writing process consolidates and deepens your understanding as well as opening up to scrutiny how you conducted the research and how valid your interpretations of the findings are. It is worth stressing that your interpretation is just that, an interpretation, and it is your job to demonstrate to the reader the validity of the research. How this is best demonstrated depends upon the intended audience as well as on the kind of research project you have conducted.

FACTORS TO CONSIDER

Writing for the intended audience

There may be various audiences for your research report, from dissertation examiners to editors and readers of journals or the participants in the research and other members of the public. Each audience will have different requirements and you need to be clear about what is expected. It may be that you will need to create different reports if you want to communicate your findings to these different audiences. Dissertation examiners put a high premium on rigour, originality and conceptual coherence, whereas the research participants or the organisation in which the research took place are likely to value accessibility, being to the point and practical outcomes.

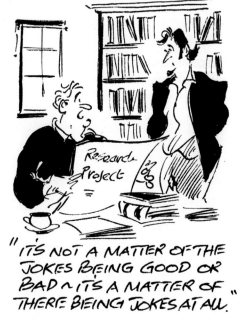

" IT'S NOT A MATTER OF THE JOKES BEING GOOD OR BAD ~ IT'S A MATTER OF THERE BEING JOKES AT ALL. "

If you are writing up your research as part of a formal course submission or for journal publication, there are likely to be very specific guidelines regarding content, style and referencing that you will have to adhere to. Whoever the intended audience, you will need to communicate why and how the research was conducted, what the findings were, how you interpreted these and what conclusions you were able to draw from this. The reader will need to make a judgement on both the significance and the trustworthiness of your findings.

> Whoever the intended audience you will need to communicate why and how the research was conducted, what the findings were, how you interpreted these and what conclusions you were able to draw from this.

Style and positioning

All audiences value clarity, good grammar and careful spellchecking. A research report may not have to be a great piece of literature, but there is no reason why you shouldn't make the report as clear and interesting as you are able. It can help if you keep in mind that you are telling a story to the audience. Most readers will appreciate a coherent report with each point leading logically to the next (not every story does this but the form is well understood). Writing in the most simple and direct language possible helps the reader follow the thread of what you are communicating. Careful use of headings, sub-headings and paragraphing will guide the reader through the report.

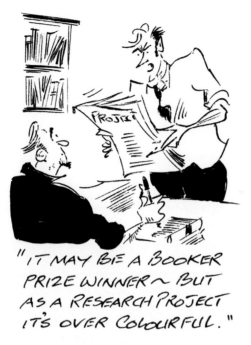

" IT MAY BE A BOOKER PRIZE WINNER ~ BUT AS A RESEARCH PROJECT IT'S OVER COLOURFUL. "

It is worth thinking about the position you are adopting as narrator of the research story to maintain consistency of style. Consider whether you are adopting the position of the detached and objective scientist, an involved advocate, a situated witness or a participant (McLeod 1994). Each of these positions implies a different way of viewing, understanding and communicating what you have found. You might ask yourself which position provides a more authentic form of expression for your research (bearing in mind your audience and formal requirements).

Don't rely exclusively on the computer for correct spelling as sometimes mistakes are real words. Changing the first letter of fat, cat, sat and mat will not show as a mistake with a computer spellchecker.

Given that the report is a document of past events, be sure to use the past tense when describing what you did or found. Pay particular attention if you import chunks of your research proposal (written in the future tense) into the final report.

Ethics of reporting

It is important to think about the political or even personal impact that your report could have on those concerned with your project. The impact could be on participants from whom you gathered data as well as on other stakeholders such as sponsors or gatekeepers who facilitated your access to the research site. If you made a commitment to participants or gatekeepers to protect their identities, then you have a moral obligation to honour this. In surveys or large-scale studies maintaining anonymity or confidentiality may be relatively easy, but in smaller-scale studies (particularly single site) this can be much more difficult. You will have to take care that disguising identities does not substantially affect the content or context of what you are saying. Readers' interpretations of critical comments about a service are likely to be influenced by what they know of the history, identity and position of those making the comments. Changing the gender, race, age or position may change the interpretation of what is written.

Genres of writing

Having identified the intended audience and clarified formal requirements and expectations set by dissertation committees or journal editors you will need to consider how best to present your research findings. A lab-based experimental study demands a somewhat different form to an ethnographic or action research study. There are conventions for all these forms and the best advice is to study the literature (with some guidance) for good and bad examples. Most medically oriented journals and academic institutions teaching health-related subjects require an impersonal formal style, written in the third person. This convention has become the standard form for reporting scientific work and the voice of science speaks with objectivity and detachment. However, though this rhetorical device may be appropriate for reporting experimental or survey work, it sits less comfortably with ethnography and other qualitative work, where the

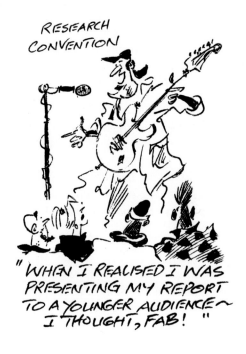

RESEARCH CONVENTION

" WHEN I REALISED I WAS PRESENTING MY REPORT TO A YOUNGER AUDIENCE — I THOUGHT, FAB! "

researcher's reflexivity is central to the analysis and validity of the research. It's a bit simplistic to refer to qualitative and quantitative genres of reporting but it is possible to differentiate some contrasting rhetorical devices used (see Table 18.1). Van Maanen (1988) usefully discusses several different styles of reporting within ethnography. These differences are rooted in the conceptual frameworks underpinning the studies (see section on conceptual frameworks in Ch. 2, General design issues). Over the last decade there has been a great deal of work exploring the validity of alternative forms of representing the findings of qualitative research (Eisner 1993, 1997). The key question to be addressed is: Given the audience you wish to communicate with and any formal conventions you must adhere to, what form will be the most congruent with the intentions, conceptual framework and methods you have used? (See section on reflexivity, objectivity and validity in Ch. 16, Analysing Qualitative Data.)

Table 18.1   Comparison of style of reporting

The realist style found in scientific reports	The relativist style found in qualitative reports
Objective	Researchers standpoint stated — subjectivity included
Written in passive voice — characteristically 3rd person	Voice of the researcher not hidden, may move from active to passive, 1st to 3rd person
Reflexivity is kept implicit or written out of the report	Reflexivity central to the validity of some qualitative reports
Conceptual framework underpinning the research methods is kept implicit. Scientific objective stance is taken as default. The conceptual framework disappears in presentation of 'the facts'	Conceptual framework underpinning the analysis is made explicit. Recognises that a range of possible frameworks can be utilised
Contextual factors mostly eliminated (only the key variables being studied are included)	Contextual factors and 'thick description' are important
Etic perspective	*Emic* perspective

CONSTRUCTING YOUR REPORT

The classic format that is a requirement for most dissertations and journals may not fit every project or audience, but the underlying logic of introducing a topic, reviewing relevant literature, describing how the study was conducted, and presenting your interpretation of the findings and your conclusion can be adapted to most projects without compromising their integrity. Perhaps there are compelling reasons why this structure should not be adhered to (for instance multi-media presentations), and if so you might

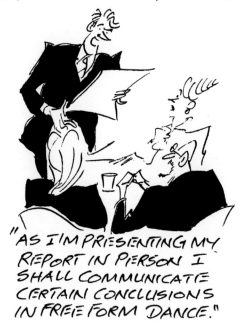

"AS I'M PRESENTING MY REPORT IN PERSON I SHALL COMMUNICATE CERTAIN CONCLUSIONS IN FREE FORM DANCE."

explore alternative options with dissertation committees, journal editors or sponsors of the report, rather than slavishly adhering to the form for its own sake. The classic format does have advantages though, not least that it is well understood by readers. Table 18.2 outlines what is normally contained in the major sections of a dissertation. Not all the following sections will be relevant in other written forms, particularly within the space constraints of a journal article. Always refer to the specific journal's guidelines for authors.

SOME ISSUES IN REPORTING QUALITATIVE DATA

There are some particular issues in writing up qualitative research that apply equally to case studies, grounded theory or ethnography.

Differentiating the raw data from your theory

Your analysis is an interplay between the raw data and your own theorising. Your reporting should differentiate between concepts and terms used by respondents (their words) and the theoretical developments you make as the

Table 18.2 Structure for reporting research within a dissertation

Section	Content
Title	The title should give a clear indication of the topic. Using a subtitle can allow more detail: for instance, a main title such as *Integrating complementary therapies* could be elaborated with a subtitle such as *a case study in general practice*.
Abstract	The abstract is a summary or synopsis of the project which rapidly allows readers to judge whether the research is relevant to them.
Preface	The preface is an opportunity to describe briefly the personal dimensions of the project, i.e. how and why the project is relevant to the researcher.
Introduction	The introduction sets the context for the research. Theoretical or practical issues that generated the research questions should be described. The aims and objectives of the research are stated. Key terms and concepts are explained. Having read the introduction the reader should have a sound understanding of why the research question is relevant and why you have adopted your chosen research strategy.
Literature review	This section is sometimes woven into an extended introduction rather than being a separate section or chapter. Wherever you decide to locate it, it is important that you demonstrate how your work relates to and builds on existing work (see Ch. 3, Reviewing the literature). The majority of the references should be current, with the exception of historical, original work. Most sources should be primary ones. They should be clearly relevant to the specific area of study. Sources whose theories or opinions conflict with those of the researcher should also be integrated or discussed.
Methods	This section should describe the research design and execution. For a journal article space limitations will probably only allow a simple summary. For a dissertation there should be sufficient detail to allow the reader to understand how and why each step of the research was conducted. Some case reports have the methods section as an appendix, if such detail would be inappropriate for the primary audience. Conceptual or theoretical considerations regarding the methodology should be discussed — for

continued over page

continued

Section	Content
	instance why you chose the specific methodology in relation to your research question. Operational aspects should also be detailed, spelling out each step taken. Employing a narrative structure leads the reader through the choices and steps taken. Depending on the design, you may need to detail aspects of: ● setting – description of research site ● participants – characteristics, numbers, how they were selected ● ethics – access to data, consent ● techniques of data collection and analysis – interview schedules, questionnaires, tests, instructions to participants, duration and number of tests or interviews, coding or scoring procedures ● validity of techniques
Findings	This is where the results are presented. Where tables and figures are used they should be clear, concise and well-labelled – a complement to rather than repetition of the text. Where statistical analysis is used to summarise data and indicate the relationships between variables, statistical methods should be described with sufficient clarity to allow the reader to verify the reported results. In quantitative studies the results are generally separated from the analyses and discussion. In qualitative studies it is not unusual to combine the findings and the analysis. The results of coding and early analysis are displayed, early analysis forming the basis for further data collection and more in-depth analysis.
Analysis/discussion	The significance of the findings is discussed and analysed in relation to theories, concepts and problems identified in the introduction and literature review. The implications for practice and further research are explored.
Conclusions	The threads are drawn together and evaluative judgements are made. There is a concise restating of implications for practice and research.
Appendices	These contain materials which would be distracting in the main text, such as proformas (questionnaires, consent forms and letters of introduction), interview extracts and technical details, and material that is either too detailed for main text or not central to understanding the research.

analyst. Your use of quotes should display how you have taken their words/concepts/theories and analysed them to develop your own theories. Take care not to collapse these together and naively accept and use respondents' theories as your own. You must go beyond recycling respondents' accounts to develop your own theoretical stance.

Using quotations

You should provide sufficient evidence for readers to make their own judgements about your theoretical developments. This does not mean you need to include complete verbatim transcripts, but if you make an analytic statement, judiciously use quotes or your own description of the data to provide evidence to ground your theory. If there is insufficient evidence presented, the reader will have no basis on which to evaluate your arguments. Your theories may appear unarguable if you present no evidence to sustain a counter argument, but they will not be more convincing for that. Another option is to fully separate the results and analysis where theory development follows presentation of the data. The issue here is that theoretical developments can appear rather dislocated from the data. A more useful approach is to work back and forth between data and theory where evidence is presented, difficulties in the data are tackled and counter evidence is put forward and discussed. The written form should describe the process of analysis — how you arrived at your theoretical insights, rather than just the insights themselves (see section 'From design to reporting' in Ch. 16, Analysing qualitative data).

NOW YOU'VE GOT THIS FAR

Having come all this way, you will need to maintain enough steam to disseminate the findings of your research to colleagues or other interested groups. If your research is to make a difference in your professional field, you need to ensure that your findings are communicated effectively. While the focus of this chapter has been on academic writing, it may be that the most effective way of reaching colleagues is through another form, such as oral presentations at conferences, collaborative groups or other forums. Presenting your work requires you to distil the essence of what you have learned. Sharing your experience and the findings of your research can be as enriching for the presenter as for the audience. Constructive criticism and feedback from face-to-face presentations can help you consolidate your understanding and refine the presentation of any final report.

Research has its highs and lows, perspiration as well as inspiration. Whatever the outcome of your particular project, the personal learning that comes from critically engaging with your subject has the potential to enrich your world of practice. The final challenge for any practitioner–researcher is to bring what you have learned through your research into the field of practice. At the very least you will have had the opportunity to develop your critical faculties and become more research aware. It may be that you learn to view some of the taken-for-granted aspects of practice with new eyes, or perhaps even make new discoveries. It is extremely rare for any one piece of research to bring about change in the whole field of practice, but a more modest aim of improving your own way of working is realistic. I wish you well in this.

References

Eisner E 1993 Forms of understanding and the future of educational research. Educational Researcher **22**(7): 5–11

Eisner E 1997 The promise and perils of alternative forms of data representation. Educational Researcher **26**(6): 4–10

McLeod A 1994 Doing counselling research. Sage, London, p 151

van Maanen J 1988 Tales from the field: on writing ethnography. University of Chicago Press, Chicago.

Index

Notes. Abbreviation: RCT = randomised controlled trial. Page numbers in *italic* refer to figures and tables.

CPI Antony Rowe
Chippenham, UK
2017-09-21 18:25